BIOGENICS:
A STEP-BY-STEP GUIDE
TO MIND AND BODY HARMONY

"Dr. Shealy has become one of the foremost pro-
ponents of Holistic Health . . . His exercises used
daily help increase energy, control pain, promote
good health."

—*Coronet*

"90 DAYS TO SELF-HEALTH emphasizes the
maintenance of health—in how-to-do-it terms . . .
Worth an honest trial for self-healing. I hope that
this book will be widely read."
    —*Journal of the American Society of Psychosomatic
    Dentistry and Medicine*

"A readable, commonsense guide to controlling
reactions to stress . . . Will enrich personal health."
    —*Body Forum*

Bantam Books by C. Norman Shealy, M.D.

90 DAYS TO SELF-HEALTH
OCCULT MEDICINE CAN SAVE YOUR LIFE

90 DAYS TO SELF- HEALTH

C. NORMAN SHEALY, M.D.

BANTAM BOOKS · TORONTO · NEW YORK · LONDON

*This low-priced Bantam Book
has been completely reset in a type face
designed for easy reading, and was printed
from new plates. It contains the complete
text of the original hard-cover edition.*
NOT ONE WORD HAS BEEN OMITTED.

90 DAYS TO SELF-HEALTH
*A Bantam Book / published by arrangement with
The Dial Press*

PRINTING HISTORY

*Dial Press edition published February 1977
4 printings through February 1978
Bantam edition / July 1978*

We appreciate permission to reproduce portions of:
Holmes, T. H., and Rabe, R. H. The social readjustment
rating scale. *Journal of Psychosomatic Research* 11 (1967):
213–218.
Masters, Roy. *How Your Mind Can Keep You Well*. Los
Angeles: Foundation Books, 1972.
Clemmons, Thomas Elbert. *Relaxation and Meditation*. West
Palm Beach, Florida: Waldemar Argow, 1976.

*Bantam Books are published by Bantam Books, Inc. Its trade-
mark, consisting of the words "Bantam Books" and the por-
trayal of a bantam, is registered in the United States Patent
Office and in other countries. Marca Registrada. Bantam
Books, Inc., 666 Fifth Avenue, New York, New York 10019.*

PRINTED IN THE UNITED STATES OF AMERICA

Contents

Foreword

At a 1975 conference called "Future Directions in Health Care: The Dimensions of Medicine" sponsored jointly by the Blue Cross Association, the Rockefeller Foundation, and the University of California Health Policy Program, a number of participants emphasized the role of the individual in a holistic approach to medical care and to health. Patients must begin to change, they maintained, from passive recipients of medical care to active self-responsible participants; otherwise our goal of developing an adequate national health system cannot be realized. Good medical care costs so much that a sizable portion of our population cannot afford it. This is partly due to the fact that at present the burden of "curing" disease and maintaining health is loaded almost entirely on the doctor. Increasingly this burden of responsibility must be shared by the patient. Helping to overcome the present bind in providing medical care by enhancing the individual's powers of self-regulation is a major purpose of this book.

Dr. Shealy outlines specific ways in which a person can take an active role in recovering from disease and in maintaining health. As a practicing physician he is concerned with what works, whatever the theory, and over the years he has assembled a battery of training methods which patients (and non-patients too) can use to improve their state of health. He does not claim to have invented all these techniques, but has modified them in various ways, according to his experience with patients, so as to maximize results. He presents here the distillation and synthesis of those self-regulation techniques he has found to be most effective.

These techniques are often successful even with patients who have suffered constant pain for many years. Such pain involves a psychological state as well as a physical state, though this is usually not recognized by patients. In fact, the overall state of health and disease in the nation involves both psychological and physiological factors. If it is true, as many physicians believe, that 50 per cent to 80 per cent of human diseases are psychosomatic (diseases that result from chronic physiological response to psychological stress), then it must also be true that a large fraction of the relief from disease can be initiated and directed from the psychological domain. In the training procedures outlined in this book the first task is to develop an *idea* of what you want the body to do—how you want the body to behave. Second, the idea (or visualization) must be coupled with *desire* for change. And third, the trainee must *willfully persevere* until the idea and desire become facts in physiological function and structure. These steps result in a consciously directed change toward psychosomatic health, in contradistinction to an unconscious slide toward psychosomatic disease.

This way of handling a medical problem may not seem possible to the uninformed person, but the logic is inescapable. If you can produce an ulcer by reacting to stress, then you can heal that same ulcer by changing your reaction. It must be admitted, of course, that in general it is the innate normal tendency of the body to move toward health that heals the ulcer—*if* the patient learns to modify stress-related reactions. Then the body has a chance to correct itself.

We must also admit there is nothing wrong with stress itself. Stress, in fact, is an essential ingredient of a joyful life. The stress of skiing down a mountain, for example, is felt as pleasure. The heart beats faster, blood pressure increases, and it is "great to be alive." But if the physiological accelerations associated with skiing do not reverse at the end of the run, we are in trouble. A temporary acceleration is natural and good, but a permanent (chronic) response can be deadly.

The problem, then, is not stress as much as the reaction to stress, and *that reaction can be to a large extent self chosen.* Through the training methods presented here we can learn to control the effects of stress and live better lives.

Our health care system is now beginning to change significantly. Holistically inclined medical doctors are becoming teachers and advisors. These physicians use surgery and drugs when necessary, but they have an important function in teaching patients how to integrate all aspects of health. This includes diet and exercise for the body, and mental and emotional exercises for the mind. "Body doctors" and "mind doctors," as isolated narrow-focus practitioners, represent only sections of medicine. Regardless of specialization, the holistic physician treats the whole patient and is concerned with body-mind-spirit synthesis. The holistic physician helps the patient achieve self-mastery and the patient ceases to be a passive victim of health problems. Self-regulation becomes an ingredient of good health.

This is what Dr. Shealy's book is about.

Elmer E. Green, Ph.D.
Director, Voluntary Controls Porgram,
Menninger Foundation
Topeka, Kansas
October 21, 1976

Personal Acknowledgments

Invariably, a book is a collection of the efforts of many different people. In writing this book, for instance, I have consulted hundreds of authors in my study of the mental exercises. Of these, particular acknowledgment is due Dr. and Mrs. Elmer Green, who introduced the most important health concept of this century— autogenic feedback. Without their lead, I could never have developed my version, Biogenics®. I am also particularly grateful to Dr. and Mrs. Green, Dr. Lindsay Jacob, and Dr. Robert Leichtman for their invaluable critiques of an early version of this work, and to many other colleagues who have added to and subtracted from the manuscript. Their assistance notwithstanding, I assume full responsibility for all statements made and all conclusions drawn.

My patients have provided me with the experience in using the techniques presented here, the success of which has encouraged me to present them to a wider audience.

Sonja Schrag, my research assistant, has contributed generously to the efforts of organizing the information; and I particularly appreciate the advice of my editor, Joyce Engelson, whose insights led to my rewriting the material to make it more useful to the reader.

Very special thanks are due my secretary, Kathleen Althoff, and my family for their patience through months of writing and rewriting.

A more technical version of this book has been submitted to the Humanistic Psychology Institute as part of my work toward a doctoral degree in psychology.

Preface

Biogenics®—a word meaning origin of life—is an elaborate system of mental exercises designed to help you learn to regulate your own body functioning at will.

This book outlines that system, developed in working with over 1,300 patients and in a number of clinical research projects, combining biofeedback, autogenic training, auto-suggestion, some Gestalt psychology, and psychosynthesis, which are increasingly used psychological techniques. It is designed as a practical, enjoyable workbook providing a three-month program for enhancing one's health. Reading it without participating in its exercises, however, will not accomplish that goal. The mental and physical exercises must be practiced. Regular daily schedules and commitment to an exercise routine will pay many dividends over the rest of your life.

In undertaking the self-regulatory techniques discussed here, readers should realize that they are designed to help maintain good general health, and, in some cases, to help correct a physiological abnormality. In certain illnesses, however, these Biogenics exercises should be undertaken only under medical supervision, particularly in cases of asthma, epilepsy, high blood pressure, active peptic ulcer, and emotional illness, especially severe neurosis, psychoneurosis, psychosis, and depression. It is essential that those readers suffering such problems seek competent medical supervision, diagnosis, and treatment. Indeed, if you develop any new symptom, do not try to treat it yourself—*seek medical care.*

Use the techniques in this book to help restore balance and then to maintain it; such balance among the physical, mental, emotional, and spiritual factors of our lives is essential. Each of these aspects of our health is equally important. One may work at perfecting only one or another of the elements, but the truly healthy person integrates—balances—all four with genuine love and compassion for others.

90 DAYS
TO SELF-HEALTH

readout of your ... level and then
... mentally detu... ... want to read...
... What you ... ... of your bod...
... our ultimately ... ... changes in ...
... ly will.
...creasingly, what ... ... been discovered is

ONE

Health, Stress, and Relaxation

Most people will agree:/Health is the most important aspect of life, and without it, little else matters. Yet in spite of the enormous sums spent in trying to *regain* one's health, most people spend very little time, effort, or money *maintaining* their most valuable asset.

Nevertheless, we know that health can be assisted by a variety of simple techniques. To focus attention on what influences health/it is worthwhile examining the major barrier to health: stress.

Is there anyone who has never experienced stress? It is unlikely that any living organism can avoid it; hardly a day passes that we don't feel at least one stressful negative emotion. Late for work? Driving in traffic? Then there are taxes, political problems, war, inflation, death, cancer, crime. Just read any newspaper, listen to the radio, or worst of all, watch television, and you've had a good strong dose of stress. We are bombarded constantly by "newsworthy" items designed to arouse our emotions. Even advertisements, which urge you to want items that may be financially out of reach, cause uneasiness and stress. In short/unless you live a protected life as a virtual hermit on some island paradise, stress is part of life—unfortunately for many, a very large part.

1

Stress itself is difficult to define, partly because it is an abstract, subjective term and hence can mean different things to different people: A situation that one person finds stressful might be considered less so or even not at all by another. Then, too, the term *stress* can apply to many conditions—some completely opposite to others. Even intensely joyful situations can be stressful; for instance, a person might be as stressed by the sudden inheritance of a sum of money as by the sudden loss of it!

Apparently the element of stress common to all types is the demand to adjust to a different situation or condition. Medical research has shown that as varied as stress-producing situations may be—and regardless of whether they are pleasant or unpleasant—the human body responds with similar biochemical changes—even if that demand is merely a behavioral one.

In one major pathology textbook, *Reaction to Injury* (1945), Dr. Wiley Forbus, the author, wisely reasoned that all illness, or disease, if you prefer, is a reaction to stress. Emotional reactions constitute a major portion of our stresses today.

Anger and fear create such intense stress that health is more seriously threatened by those emotions than almost all other influence. Dr. Arnold Hutschnecker in his book *The Will to Live* says, "We know that a man who puts a bullet into his brain does so with the full intention of killing himself. It is not so obvious that another man may be killing himself just as surely—even though unconsciously—by way of illness."

Anxiety is not an invention of the latter part of the twentieth century; it has existed throughout recorded history and is evident from the folk tales preceding even written record. Fear of natural catastrophe must have been greater 3,000 years ago than it is today, but today modern communications magnify the pressure of every unhappy event. *Good* news is not news, so it claims little space in television, radio, or newsprint. We are constantly presented with the threats of financial disaster, war, atomic annihilation, pollution, crime, and starvation. Television ads proclaim the problems of

mankind every hour of the day. We are reminded of
the generation gap, of the divorce explosion, of noise
pollution, *ad nauseam*.

And compounding the ill effects of those grim
warnings, the roots of family life have been truly torn
from their historical garden. The recent facility of trans-
portation has produced an itinerant society in which
many families change homes more than once a year.
The incidence of serious psychological distress increases
with the frequency of moving, which prior to World
War II was considerably less common. The overall
emotional stability of an extended family so common in
the last century has been replaced not only by restless
mobility but by anonymity, and the necessity to crowd
into greater and greater metropolitan complexes. Even
rats develop serious reactions to stress when over-
crowded. And *emotional stress, like physical stress, low-
ers resistance to disease.*

Despite the vast sums of money spent on medical
treatment in America, the number of people who are ill
remains high. All the miracle drugs and heroic surgical
advances notwithstanding, the health of humanity has
not greatly improved. Infectious diseases have been replaced as the greatest cause of death by cancer and
hardening of the arteries, which, in the opinion of many,
are largely diseases of stress. Often patients come to
their doctors with problems of high blood pressure,
gastritis, chest pain, or constipation, and the physician
diagnoses the disease as "functional" or psychosomatic,
which means there is no physical abnormality to explain
the symptoms. Patients are told it's "just nerves," and
tranquilizers are prescribed. But the question of what
caused the condition is not answered. And why is it that
billions of tranquilizers later we are not a healthier nation?

On the other hand, why is it that in an epidemic
of infectious illness only a certain percentage of people
contract the disease and even fewer die of it? Why do
some people seem immune to sickness?

In response to all those questions, we turn repeatedly to the answer, *emotional stress.* Anxiety and

other manifestations of emotional distress most often are not serious problems with some morbid hidden meaning; they are simple *overreactions* to ordinary events. But anger, frustration, depression, hatred, anxiety, fear, and guilt are real stresses. They create physical dis-ease. They weaken the system of immunity. They stimulate the body to produce excess adrenalin and cortisone, and, in general, they upset the homeostasis—the balance—of the various functions of the body. This dysautonomia, disturbance of the automatic functioning mechanism of the body, results in most symptoms and diseases. Stress also leads to tremendous fatigue; it wears us out. No one can avoid experiencing stress, but everyone does have the capacity to regulate the *reactions* to stress, and to avoid having the stress lead to severe anxiety and more serious emotional distress.

As Dr. Hutschnecker has said, also in *The Will to Live,* "Anxiety is a whisper of danger from the unconscious; whether the danger is real or imagined, the threat to health is real; depression is a partial surrender to death."

Unfortunately, the entire concept of psychosomatic illness has been felt by many to imply some willful scheming on the part of the patient, some sinister manipulation or some form of malingering. Nothing could be less true. Most patients given insight into their stress are eager to come to grips with their reactions which, left untended, can become destructive. The psychosomatic symptom is really brought on through lack of knowledge about how to balance the extremes of emotion. Even well-adjusted people are exposed to such distress and need to regulate its effect upon the body.

Colitis, tachycardia (racing heart), high blood pressure, asthma, hives, most skin rashes, most fainting, blushing, sweating, trembling, and most instances of dizziness are only a few of the common illnesses or symptoms which are reactions to emotional stress. Depression, which might seem to be the opposite of stress, also brings about powerful physiological changes in the hormone system. Without your exercising any conscious control over it, your autonomic nervous system and all your body functions react vigorously to both stress and depression.

Since the hormones you produce normally remain within very narrow levels, when you experience stress of any kind, alteration of the normal levels of many of those hormones quickly causes trouble. When the body is stressed, it prepares for fight or flight, and needs, in order to function, additional cortisone. It needs additional adrenalin. It needs additional thyroid hormone. Estrogen and testosterone levels are then lowered. So when you are put in a stressful situation, whether it is emotional or physical—and the body can't always distinguish between the two—you start producing changes in the levels of those hormones. If the stress goes on long enough, the basic metabolism of the body may become quite disturbed. And after the stress is resolved, the body doesn't always settle back down to that nice normal level that it usually maintains.

The primary purpose of this book is to help you become aware that you can alter all those body functions with mental self-control.

Most people accept the fact that a peptic ulcer is a disease of stress. Emotional stress commonly leads to gastric irritation, beginning with a raw, empty feeling that something is wrong in the abdomen. Then there is the pain, which is relieved by milk or food, and aggravated by coffee, cigarettes, alcohol, and aspirin, all things that either increase the intensity of stress or whose acidity eats away at tender tissues. If the ulcer gets bad enough, it will erode a blood vessel and bleed; and if it gets to bleeding enough, you go into shock.

Now, if it's true that emotional distress can eat a hole in your stomach, it can do all kinds of other things as well. Almost every illness has this mixture of purely physical factors—things you can see, like a knife wound or a fractured bone—plus certain chemical factors such as metabolic changes occurring within the body. Almost every disease has associated with it the alterations occurring in the body as the result of the emotional distress that either preceded the illness, accompanied it, or came on because of it.

All of us have physical weak spots, and all of us

have emotional weak spots. For instance, some whole families have a tendency toward diabetes. If you were to look at all the members of that family—cousins, aunts, uncles, and so on—you would find a much higher percentage of people with diabetes than in a family that doesn't have the tendency.

We are also born with relative differences in emotional weakness. You see this in children from their earliest days. There are many people who seem to be born with an absolutely happy personality and there is almost nothing you can do to upset them; they are happy and gay no matter what happens. And there are others who are exactly the opposite: No matter what happens, they are unhappy. You can give such a person a million dollars and he would say, "Oh, well, the government will take practically all of it anyhow."

People have also been tested according to environmental influences—early training and the like—and found to have emotional weaknesses in relation to special things that happen. Some people, for instance, would become terribly distressed if you accused them of being homosexual, while others march in the streets proclaiming their homosexuality. These are indications of relative emotional strengths or weaknesses, if you will, and not a judgment of either kind of person.

Probably you are already well aware of such differences in emotional tendencies; you know that some people if threatened with the loss of their job would say, "Thank God, now I can do something else," while others would go into a severe depression from which they might have trouble recovering. Others would develop a peptic ulcer, and still others might even come down with rheumatoid arthritis. And consider cancer. Even though we know of the existence of chemical and physical factors, psychologists have also known for many years that a patient who develops a flagrant cancerous process often has a distinct personality. Such a person usually tends to be too passive and says, in effect, to the rest of the world, "Go ahead, run over me. I don't care, everything is going to be all right." Putting on that kind of face for the world is an emotional stress. In fact, to some extent, the sweetest people die of can-

cer. They are just too nice. They are not standing up
for themselves on the social scene, nor are they using
their own immune mechanisms to fight for their own
physical well-being. In fact, statistics have shown that,
most often, a major loss of love, such as divorce or
death, has occurred within 18 months previous to the
onset of the disease.

But there are positive implications to such a notion as well. Dr. Carl Simonton of Texas (Simonton,
Carl and Stephanie: Belief Systems and Management of
the Emotional Aspects of Malignancy, *J. Transpersonal
Psychology*, 7:29–47, 1975) has demonstrated beyond
any reasonable doubt that emotions can affect cancer,
even leading to its disappearance. In a test of over 300
cases, he taught the patients techniques for manipulating
mentally their immune mechanisms. The results were
that 98 percent of those who practiced the techniques
only 15 minutes three times a day experienced a shrink-
ing of their cancers; those patients in his series who did
not died of their cancer. All his patients presumably
had the same underlying physical problems. Their cancers had been induced by viruses and/or chemicals. Yet
there was a difference in what happened to the process,
presumably based on what they did about it once started.

Research done over the past half century by the
greatest living Canadian scientist, Dr. Hans Selye, has
indicated that stress creates a definite biological syndrome. After noting that most diseases, regardless of
which ones, have in common certain readily evident
signs, for example, loss of appetite and weight, he found
in his experimentation more objective proof of disease
damage: enlargement of the adrenal glands, shrinkage
of the lymphatic structure, and the appearance of gastrointestinal ulcers. Dr. Selye theorized that all these symptoms—the same ones even among different diseases—
were all part of the body's alarm reaction to the disease
invasion.

He also found that if the onslaught continues, the
body adjusts and goes into what he called the "stage of
resistance" or "adaptation" during which the body affects normality. But finally, if the stress does not cease,
the body becomes exhausted and debilitated from the

wear and tear of constant readjustment. This three-stage process Selye called the General Adaptation Syndrome, or GAS.

The processes of the GAS include numerous biochemical changes, one of the most widely known of which is the secretion of adrenalin. In addition, stress excites the hypothalamus, which causes the pituitary, the small gland just below it, to increase secretion of the hormone ACTH. That hormone, in turn, stimulates the adrenal cortex to produce corticoids, some of which cause atrophy (wasting away) of the thymus. Through this chain reaction, stress can affect metabolism and body weight. Various ailments are initiated as a result of the derangement in the secretion of these hormones, such as ulcers and stomach upsets, headaches, certain allergies and sinus attacks, and cardiovascular diseases.

Of course, other factors enter into determining the degree of damage done by stress. The way one responds to stress can be attributed in part to such factors as age, sex, and genetic background, or to external conditions such as diet or medical treatment. Apparently, those factors make the differences among the levels of stress that can be tolerated by different people before disease sets in.

The biochemical mechanisms that work to counteract stress and to maintain the normal balance of the system are numerous and complex, but, in general, they act either to create a state of tolerance to stress-producing agents or to destroy the agents. Although those reactions are usually appropriate and necessary, sometimes they are inappropriate or excessive. This kind of systemic miscalculation can in itself cause disease. Allergies are a case in point: In an allergic reaction the body is reacting to invasion of foreign particles, that is, the allergens, much more aggressively than is really necessary, considering the dangers the allergens represent. So, you see, even the body's natural reactions to stress are not above error.

But, though reacting to stress is not only unavoidable but a very necessary element of life, it is possible to avoid *overreactions* by first understanding the workings of stress. Then it's necessary to establish a philosophy of life and a style of living to allow for your adjusting more readily to the inevitable stressful situations that go along with being alive.

Rest assured that it is definitely possible to regulate your reaction to stress. And the more you learn to control such reactions, the happier and healthier you should be. It is essential, of course, that you always seek proper medical care for any real illness. Self-diagnosis or treatment of any symptom or disease is not recommended. This book is designed to teach you techniques that you may use to come to grips with yourself to avoid unnecessary wear and tear on your body and mind with the stresses of life. As stated previously, if you have asthma, an active peptic ulcer, angina pectoris, epilepsy, or uncontrolled high blood pressure, or are under psychiatric treatment, you should not consider undertaking the mental and physical exercises in this book except with the approval of your own physician.

This book is not oriented toward the treatment of any of the stresses mentioned, but rather toward the avoidance of the ultimate and most severe stress—emotional distress. We cannot teach you to avoid the stressful situations. It is difficult, for example, for anyone to alter the frustrating bureaucratic procedures that face most of us at work. But we can teach you how to *cope with* the stress caused by the world in which we live and work.

In general, I believe that *every* human being should practice Biogenics. These relaxation-balancing techniques are safe and health promoting and will not interfere with any standard medical therapy. Indeed they will assist your physician's treatment program by helping you minimize the distress of many life events.

Let us first consider the relative intensity of a variety of stresses.

THE STRESS OF ADJUSTING TO CHANGE

Psychiatrists Thomas H. Holmes and Richard H. Rabe of the University of Washington Medical School have evaluated the relative distress of various events and produced the following "social readjustment scale,"

rating certain stressful situations on a scale of 1 to 100.*
As your total score increases, so does the likelihood of
illness.

Event	Scale of Impact
Death of spouse	100
Divorce	73
Marital separation	65
Jail term	63
Death of close family member	63
Personal injury or illness	53
Marriage	50
Fired at work	47
Marital reconciliation	45
Retirement	45
Change in health of family member	44
Pregnancy	40
Sex difficulties	39
Gain of new family member	39
Business readjustment	39
Change in financial state	38
Death of close friend	37
Change to different line of work	36
Change in number of arguments with spouse	35
Mortgage over $10,000	31
Foreclosure of mortgage or loan	30
Change in responsibilities at work	29
Son or daughter leaving home	29
Trouble with in-laws	29
Outstanding personal achievement	28
Wife begins or stops work	26
Begin or end school	26
Change in living conditions	25
Revision of personal habits	24
Trouble with boss	23
Change in work hours or conditions	20
Change in residence	20
Change in schools	20
Change in recreation	19
Change in church activities	19
Change in social activities	18
Mortgage or loan less than $10,000	17

*Reproduced with permission of the authors and publisher from
T. H. Holmes and R. H. Rabe, "The Social Readjustment Rating
Scale," *Journal of Psychosomatic Research 11:* 213–218, 1967.

Event	Scale of Impact
Change in sleeping habits	16
Change in number of family get-togethers	15
Change in eating habits	15
Vacation	13
Christmas	12
Minor violations of the law	11

Looking at those first two items, it has been noted that 10 times more widows and widowers die within a year of the death of their spouses than is expected in the general population, and that divorced persons become ill during the first year after divorce 12 times as commonly as married persons. Note that even "happy" events, such as Christmas and vacations, are also stressful.

Dr. Seymour Rosenblatt of Mt. Sinai Hospital in New York City has reported that 86 percent of depressed neurotics develop significant alterations in the immune response. This may result from the marked increase in cortisone production which accompanies stress —and depression is definitely stressful.

So are even many of our daily thoughts. Have you ever called someone a pain in the neck? Or a pill? Have you ever had trouble sleeping because of worry? Have you ever said, "He (or she) makes me sick"? What about, "That'll be the death of me," or "I could have died." The many dozens of such common slang expressions emphasize our concerns with emotions and health; they also give expression to the correlation between stressful emotions and our physical well-being.

It is also important that we recognize that stress leads to muscle tension, which tends to build up over a period of months into a generalized state of altered physiology. Unchecked, this tension, through the functions of the autonomic nervous system, leads ultimately to disease.

The autonomic nervous system controls the size of the blood vessels and regulates all the inner organs, in other words, it is really what makes the body run. Theoretically, it is not under our volitional management, and to a large extent that is true. Very few people are born with the ability to exercise conscious control over the autonomic system. You probably don't even know in what part of the body that control is found, or what the control system is called. Termed the limbic system, it is in the brain and determines the functioning of the hypothalamus, and the pituitary gland, and, through these centers, in a way, everything that happens in the body.

The usefulness of understanding the interrelations of systems of organs and their ultimate regulation by the brain through hypothalamic regulation was dealt a backward blow early in this century when the American master of medicine of that time, Sir William Osler (1849–1919), proclaimed that all symptoms should be relegated to a single diagnosis. Thus, it is still more difficult today for doctors to diagnose tuberculosis and ulcerative colitis in the same patients, since they have been taught to try to diagnose only one disturbance or "syndrome." As it turns out, Osler was probably correct in a way (although most physicians today might not understand the way) if "single diagnosis" is interpreted as "reaction to stress." A case history may help:

M. A., a thirty-five-year-old housewife, told me that she was certain that her TB at the age of twenty had been the result of the severe emotional stress of subjugation by an aunt who raised her. The aunt had buried three husbands (two of whom had died of cancer) and intended that the patient never marry but remain at home to take care of her. Her constant suppression and browbeating took their toll on M. A. in the form of a case of tuberculosis, for which she was confined to a sanitarium. She begged the doctors to allow her to treat her own disease through the exercise of will, but, as she was under twenty-one, her aunt gave permission for surgery. She almost died of tuberculous pneumonia. Only after three years at the sanitarium, away from her aunt, was she able to heal herself. She then ran away to be married so that she could avoid her overbearing aunt.

A single diagnosis of M. A.'s disease would be TB, but a comprehensive view of the patient indicates that her real problem was emotional distress. Interestingly, even Osler understood that the outcome of cases of tuberculosis depended more upon "what [the patients] have in their heads than on what is in their chests." The influence of emotional stress upon the body's ability to develop natural immunity to infectious agents is probably much greater than is generally known.

COMMON EMOTION-BASED DISEASES

Although stress ordinarily leads to further weakening of the person's inherent weak spots, certain emotional disturbances do tend to affect specific organs.

For instance, inhibited or unresolved rage has a particularly adverse effect upon the heart and blood vessels, whether or not those are the patient's weak spots. Dr. Caroline Thomas at Johns Hopkins Medical School in Baltimore has carried out a continuing evaluation of 1,337 medical students, which has emphasized that excessive passivity is a trait often seen in cancer patients.* And the need to overproduce, common among peptic ulcer patients, is well known. An intense craving for love that has been frustrated or unrealized most often leads to overeating and obesity. The spastic colon patient is characterized as dependent, sensitive, anxious, guilt-ridden, resentful, and overconscientious, a fairly wide range of kinds of emotional stress. Similarly, ulcerative colitis may be an intense reaction to strong conflicts of dependency, guilt, anxiety, and the urge to accomplish in the face of deep feelings of incompetence.

As in most psychophysiological disturbances, asthma is associated with anxiety, jealousy, extreme anger, and most other forms of sudden, intense emotional upset. No single personality disturbance is characteristic in this broad-based emotionally oriented illness. Often, however, there is an intense, repressed dependence upon the mother. It has been suggested that this disease

---

*Thomas, Caroline, "Human Figure Drawing in a Prospective Study of Six Disease States," *J. of Nervous and Mental Diseases*, 161:191–199, 1975.

is especially one of an unresolved Oedipus complex. Despite findings of allergies in many types of asthmatics, the basic disturbance, even of the immune system, seems to be primarily one of emotional imbalance.

Constipation is another psychophysiological disturbance in which patients typically have a depressed, pessimistic, defeatist attitude, and feelings of rejection and being unloved.

Most patients with high blood pressure have greater or lesser problems of inhibited hostility. Such patients may suffer extreme anxiety or a sense of guilt as a result of their feelings of hostility, but, being overcontrolled and unable to express themselves, they destroy themselves instead of the objects of their anger. Society requires control of aggresssion, but if a satisfactory resolution is not achieved, a condition such as high blood pressure may ensue.

Migraine is one of the best-known psychogenic problems. These patients are often ambitious, reserved, outwardly relaxed and dignified, sensitive, and lacking in a sense of humor and in sexual adjustment. The excess compulsiveness of migraine sufferers is emphasized by one headache expert who said he always asks a female migraine patient whether she can go to bed at night without washing the dishes. If she can, then he does *not* diagnose true migraine!

Most skin disorders are some form of neurodermatitis: blushing, skin pallor, goose pimples, bristling of the hair, and excess sweating are the most widely recognized reactions to emotional stress. Eczema, itching, edema, or swelling, sudden loss of hair, psoriasis, and a variety of "allergic" rashes seem remarkably related to—you guessed it—repressed hostility, resulting in guilt and self-punishment—unconscious though it may be. Most psychiatrists consider scratching inhibited sexual excitement. Freud certainly got around!

Almost all endocrine disorders have been related to emotional distress. An overactive thyroid is one of the easiest to recognize. Sudden emotional conflict or psychic trauma is commonly found in such cases. Even physical trauma, such as an automobile accident, may precipitate the onset of an overactive thyroid.

Even so simple a symptom as fatigue is much more commonly due to mental exhaustion than to physical exertion. Boredom is a very common cause of fatigue, leading to great waste of energy. Frustration, lack of hope, lack of incentive, anxiety, and fear are all great sappers of energy.

The emotional aspects of diabetes are equally well known, although heredity and diet influences the disease as well, of course. Obesity is present in nearly 75 percent of diabetics, which in itself attests to the existence of strong emotional influences, but only 5 percent of obese patients develop diabetes. Self-pity and a desire to be taken care of, conflicting with the demands to give to others, in combination with a sudden shock of any kind, may precipitate diabetes in those predisposed to it.

The remarkable relation of rheumatoid arthritis, being an auto-immune disorder, to emotional disturbance is also well documented. The disease is often associated with hostility, rebellion, and resentment, and the guilt that accompanies such feelings. Some psychiatrists have suggested that such problems begin as a reaction to excessively restrictive parents.

Even accidents are emotionally related. Although clumsiness, fatigue, and absent-mindedness are often cited as the cause of accidents, people who have one accident are much more likely to have another than those who have never suffered an accident.

In one Connecticut study, for instance, only 3.9 percent of the drivers involved in any accident, were involved in as many as 36.4 percent of all accidents! Most accidents appear to be subconsciously motivated. When questioned, 60 percent of the participants in the study who had suffered fractures admitted to feelings of guilt and resentment toward some person at the time of the accident. Accident-prone people are often known to carry deep resentment of authority figures.

Emotional stress, in such forms as fear, anger, or guilt, is really contagious, especially to those most intimately related. Attitudes and emotions are most strongly conveyed to children, and often a lifetime of distress is set up when a child is exposed to stress in the home. Excessive expressions of fear, irritation, and anger create insecurity, fear, guilt, and depression. Under hypnotic questioning, many seriously disturbed patients have recalled devastating events of early childhood, or even infancy, events that set a pattern of continuing emotional stress and physiological imbalance. If you've read *Sybil,* the most startling example of this, you'll realize that even much less severe episodes can, in varying degrees, put a child's emotional thermostat out of order.

Human beings react to threats and symbols of danger just as strongly as to actual physical danger. Indeed, sometimes imagined or emotional threats are far more harmful than most natural catastrophes. These threats are forms of harmful stress for they imply a potentially serious danger. For instance the *threat* of rape may be more upsetting to *some* individuals than the attack. And some persons threatened with murder die from the distress.

And a given stress may be of much greater disturbance at some times than others. For instance, if an individual has had insufficient sleep he may blow his cool at the normal noise his children make, whereas if everything else is stable he may join in the funmaking.

Apparently, our most common symptom of stress is headache, most often coming from muscle tension—that is, the sustained contraction of neck muscles brought on by tension. Indeed, muscles throughout the body, representing the greatest bulk of tissue, are also responsible for many other symptoms. Backaches and leg and arm pains, for example, are often due to chronic muscle tension, called "armoring" by the great psychiatrist, Wilhelm Reich. Dissatisfaction and resentment, fear, and almost any type of restrained emotions all lead to body armoring, or tense muscles.

To this point I have emphasized the effects of stress—or distress—in producing disease. It is important to recognize that I am not ignoring all the other major factors that contribute to illness. Consider the following complicated interrelationships.

We generally classify diseases as congenital, vascular, immunological, environmental, infectious, neoplastic, chemical, degenerative, or emotional. I'll define these terms, give some common examples of diagnoses fitting these categories, and then demonstrate that such simplistic pigeonholing is quite inadequate to explain totally any disease process.

Congenital: Referring to a condition with which one is born, which exists through heredity or the health of the mother during pregnancy. Well-known congenital diseases include cerebral palsy, some types of muscular dystrophy, hydrocephalus ("water on the brain"), many congenital heart diseases ("blue baby," for example). In addition to being the root of such diseases, however, genetic weaknesses *predispose* individuals to many illnesses, which, after a buildup of stress, come on later in life. Cancer, diabetes, rheumatoid arthritis, and allergies represent such problems.

Vascular: Having to do with disorders of the blood vessels or blood elements. Hardening of the arteries, heart attacks, strokes, blood clots, anemia, high blood pressure are well-known illnesses affecting the blood elements. In addition, however, the integrity of the vascular system largely influences most other diseases. For instance, in diabetes the blood vessels are often damaged, leading to many of the further complications of the disease.

Immunological: Arising from disturbances of the immune system, and causing such diseases as hay fever, asthma, allergies, rheumatoid arthritis, cancer, multiple sclerosis, and infections. Blood proteins called antibodies, white blood cells, the spleen, and lymph nodes are prominent organs responsible for maintaining proper immunity or protection from foreign proteins such as bacteria.

Environmental: We all are familiar with the meaning of this term, and every disease is intimately related to a variety of environmental factors—air, water, chemicals, and so on, as well as the general emotional climate of one's home life. Accidents or trauma represent the extremes of the causes of environmental illnesses. Miner's, or farmer's, lung is also a well-known environmental disease.

Infectious: Referring to a condition arising from

the presence of bacteria, viruses, fungi, or parasites. All have been implicated as causative factors in a wide variety of illnesses, and for many of the most serious infectious diseases, inoculations have been developed to help one develop immunity. But one's congenital strength, immune system, vascular network, and environment all must be evaluated in determining "cause."

Neoplastic: Referring to a disorder caused by the presence of a tumor, either benign or malignant (cancerous), the latter kind being well known as the third most common cause of death. But congenital, environmental, immunological, infectious, and vascular factors all play roles in the development and growth of tumors.

Chemical: Having to do with a harmful imbalance of the innumerable substances in our bodies necessary to maintain life. Although they cross the line into environmental diseases, lead poisoning and disorders caused by the toxicity of a wide variety of sprays and additives to which we are exposed are chemical diseases. Internal chemical disorders also include dozens of illnesses such as diabetes and myasthenia gravis. In such disorders, diet is obviously of crucial importance.

Degenerative: Slowly advancing, never retreating, wear-and-tear type problems. But trauma and chemical influences and immunological, infectious, vascular, and congenital factors interact to produce these diseases, such as osteoarthritis.

Emotional or psychological: The mental illnesses, generally understood as being restricted to the more serious or psychotic disorders such as schizophrenia. But even here environmental, congenital, and chemical aspects are strongly evident. And the broadest view must include the effects of emotional stress on the body as a whole—the psychosomatic illnesses.

One of the greatest problems in American medicine has been the pigeonholing of diseases into small etiologic categories when, in fact, every disease affects the entire function of body and mind. In reality we should assess in diagnosis the relative contribution of each of the above factors in every patient. Whenever possible, every conceivable influence should be weighed and balanced to the best of our ability for effective diagnosis and treatment.

It is really unfortunate that the words "emotional" and "psychosomatic" have been used to describe illnesses, most of which are actually diseases of stress. Now doesn't that term sound better than "emotional"? And the notion of "stress" is certainly more inclusive than "emotion." Physical stress, for instance, is just as great a strain as chemical, electrical, or emotional stress.

Now consider the remarkably complex interreactions among some of those illnesses mentioned earlier, recognizing that a single classification cannot be used. Infections require the presence of a microorganism: bacteria, fungus, virus, protozoa, or such. However, these organisms far outnumber all other forms of life, and they are omnipresent. Everyone has a relative resistance to infectious agents, partly congenital and markedly influenced by the immunological power of the body. This resistance is related to the adequacy of blood supply (vascular) and lowered when one has a tumor (neoplastic) or where there has been injury (trauma). It is significantly affected by chemicals (diet, drugs, poisons, and so on) and most directly altered by emotional distress. Depression, for instance, alters the immunity of the body making it more prone to infections. The same is true of other emotional stresses.

It is of considerable interest that the greatest pathologist of all time, Rudolf Virchow (1821–1902), reported that he felt that germs "seek their natural habitat," that is, that diseased tissue, rather than being the "cause" of the disease, actually attracts it—just as mosquitoes seek stagnant water but do not make fresh water stagnant.

Cancer, too, is related to such factors as the stability of the immune system, trauma, chemicals, infectious agents (some viruses), blood supply, congenital susceptibility, and—emotions. As mentioned earlier, most cancer patients have the clinical onset of their illness within 18 months of some major emotional trauma. For instance, one mother developed widespread breast cancer within months of her son's suicide. Similar relationships of the disease to divorce, deaths of loved ones, and so on are much too common to be ignored. And one of the most striking cases of the response of cancer to emotional *rebalancing* through the exercises presented later in this book is the case of a lovely 50-year-old widow who, after two and a half weeks of practice, suddenly became free of pain from widespread breast cancer which had invaded her bones. She not only learned to control her pain, but has become fully active, and there no longer exists any clinical evidence of cancer.

I could give examples of almost any illness you wish to mention in which the problem has been cleared up by the use of Biogenic techniques. I could give you an equal number of examples in which the problem has been aggravated badly by a person's negative emotions. I therefore conclude that *if all these symptoms and diseases can be caused by emotional distress, then by controlling emotional excesses mentally, one can learn to control most symptoms and most disease processes.*

A remarkable example among my patients is the case of a sixty-year-old depressed widow with a five-year history of severe rheumatoid arthritis which had failed to respond to aspirin, cortisone, or gold shots, the latter having left her bone-marrow depressed. I explained to her the need for a six-month program of self-regulatory practice after our two weeks of instructions, but after only ten days she angrily went home because she was no better. Three weeks later she nearly died of a bleeding peptic ulcer—real proof that she was suffering stress—and had to have two-thirds of her stomach removed. But three months later, all her arthritis and ulcer symptoms disappeared when she suddenly eloped with a new-found lover!

But even where no severe stress is evident, it is wise to suspect a possible role emotions could be playing. Take, for instance, the case of an apparently well-adjusted seventy-year-old widow who had suffered moderate, active rheumatoid arthritis for twenty-six years, with little therapeutic benefit from aspirin, cortisone, or gold. After only one month of Biogenics, she lost all symptoms of active arthritis. Apparently, even though she was not suffering severe emotional distress, the emotional rebalancing effected with autogenic practice strengthened her own healing abilities. How many other "auto-immune" disorders might respond in the same way?

Diabetes is a fascinating and complex disorder of sugar metabolism, influenced by hereditary tendencies, trauma (stress), infections, and chemicals (diet, cortisone). The disease leads to certain degenerative changes especially in blood vessels, but is often exacerbated by emotional distress. For example, one widow who had had a very unhappy marriage became so overwhelmed with guilt after her husband's death that she developed both high blood pressure and severe diabetes. By the same token, an eighty-five-year-old woman with insulin-dependent diabetes and angina pectoris (hardening of the arteries of the heart) overcame both illnesses by developing a positive attitude and engaging in vigorous physical exercise—running 5 miles a day!

Rheumatoid arthritis is another striking example of complex interreactions. There is a definite hereditary influence and an alteration of the immune system (the problem is partly an immunity to oneself!), and the condition is made worse by trauma and may also be related to streptococcal infections. It often involves the vascular system and leads to degenerative joint changes. It is definitely influenced by chemicals (cortisone and aspirin) and is always aggravated by emotional distress. Indeed, depressed individuals develop a positive "rheumatoid factor."

Peptic ulcer is an illness widely recognized as a reaction to emotional stress. And yet it is certainly influenced by heredity, chemicals (diet, cortisone, aspirin, and other drugs), and infections. But as we've emphasized, the best way to avoid or to treat peptic ulcer is to achieve emotional harmony in one's daily life.

One of the most controversial illnesses is hardening of the arteries, which has been extensively argued to be related to diet. Homogenization of milk, coffee, animal fats, sugar, vitamin E, vitamin C, cadmium–zinc balance, salt, bulk (fiber), and a whole host of other dietary factors have been implicated. But heredity, physical exercise, high blood pressure, diabetes, smoking, sexual activity, body weight, and hormones all have a role to play. But most significant, perhaps, is personality. The Type A personality—tense, hard-driving, never-relaxed, who often smokes and drinks coffee to excess—is a perfect candidate for heart attack. One typical Type A man had his first heart attack at age fifty, 15 months after a divorce and one month after remarriage. He was 20 pounds overweight but refused to reduce or to give up either his two to three packs of cigarettes a day or his five to six cups of coffee a day. One of my professors, Dr. Sam Martin, softened the distress of his family with the comment, "Every adult has a right to choose how he dies." The third heart attack, at age fifty-four, was fatal. Four brothers with similar personalities and weight and smoking problems all died in their early fifties, but one other brother, a calm Type B, thin and physically active, remains healthy at the age of seventy.

Allergies, which are known to cause hay fever, asthma, and many other diseases, are a particularly interesting problem. There is a strong hereditary influence, they are often triggered by infections and allergic patients suffer more frequent infections, but numerous questions regarding their cause and treatment remain unanswered. It is known that chemicals, such as cortisone, histamine, and various substances to which individuals are allergic, including foods, are significantly related, and that there also occurs a disturbance in the immune system. Emotions play a decisive role in both acute attacks and the chronicity of the symptoms.

Even though the major factors responsible for glaucoma are not well known, it has been demonstrated that eye pressures may be quite effectively controlled by allowing the patient to see a constant record of the pressures as they are recorded, which is one form of biofeedback.

Endocrine or hormonal disorders, especially an overactive thyroid and disturbances of the menstrual cycle, are among the most significant psychological stress reactions. Even fertility is affected. Consider, for instance, the well-known high incidence of conception shortly after adoption among women who have had a problem conceiving. Hyperthyroidism is very often seen shortly after pregnancy, which produces chemical, physical, and emotional stress, or trauma, an auto accident, for instance, or the death of a loved one.

Epilepsy is a peculiar illness, most commonly of "unknown" cause. And yet it is known to be influenced by heredity (twice as many epileptics are found in the family of an epileptic as in that of a non-epileptic), infections, trauma, blood supply (hemorrhages or clotting of blood vessels), tumors (about one-third of adults with fresh onset of epilepsy have a tumor), and chemistry (even excess salt or water can lead to a seizure in a particularly susceptible individual). Emotional stress is strongly influential in the frequency of seizures. I know of at least one marriage that broke up largely because of the frequency of seizures during sexual intercourse. Apparently, even pleasant stress can trigger problems!

Spastic colon, that is, alternating attacks of diarrhea and constipation, is most often the result of chronic anxiety, influenced significantly by diet (chemicals) and probably by many other factors. The symptoms can largely be controlled by Biogenics.

High blood pressure most often is idiopathic, that is, of unknown cause. It is influenced by chemicals (diet, salt, cortisone, zinc, and cadmium), level of blood sugar, heredity, infections, trauma (stress), and some tumors (especially of the adrenal glands) and is very responsive to emotions. Most patients with mild high blood pressure have an automatic increase of 10 to 30 points in blood pressure upon entering a doctor's office. Self-regulatory mental exercises usually reduce blood pressure 10 percent even during the first sessions, and continuing practice may remove the need for drugs to relieve the condition.

Psychiatrists have reported for a long time that if you relieve one symptom in a chronically anxious patient, something else will crop up, some other autonomic dysfunction will occur. When dealing with any imbalanced state, it is important to recognize the potential for developing alternative symptoms and ultimately other disease processes, and it's one of the reasons that we emphasize so strongly the fact that you should work to put your whole body, mind, emotions, and spirit in tune.

Furthermore, the autonomic nervous system is so diffusely represented within the body that it's like God. It's really everywhere. Its job is the universal balancing mechanism of the body. Outside the body cavities, in the arms and legs, and on the surface of the skin, the autonomic nervous system travels to its destination by riding piggyback on the coattails of the blood vessels. It doesn't have discrete nerve trunks or nerves that wander off by themselves. Most individuals know about the sciatic nerve—that's a nerve trunk, a specific pathway, with lots of branches, but nevertheless a distinct general direction. The autonomic nervous system, which is outside the spinal canal and the body cavities, doesn't have nerves like that. The nerves are wrapped around the blood vessels, and they travel wherever the blood vessels travel.

The primary function of the autonomic system in these outer parts of the body is to control the circulation of the blood. These nerves actually manipulate the blood vessels. They make them smaller or larger, depending upon the state of excitement. If the autonomic nervous system is not under stress, then the blood vessels are normally dilated. If you become relaxed beyond normal, they dilate further. If you become uptight, they constrict, making your hands and feet cold, and often, at the same time.

In addition to these normal actions of the autonomic nervous system (and lots of others that we haven't related here), when the body is physically damaged, the autonomic nerves try to regrow just as other nerves try to regrow, and you begin to get some anatomically mixed-up nerves. Often they don't grow along the same blood vessels as before, or the blood vessel may have been cut or torn and have regrown into some part of the body where they did not normally go. So an autonomic nerve fiber that is supposed to be curling around a specific blood vessel may find itself stuck to bone or in a piece of scar. When that occurs, the information sent reflexly into the nervous system will be inappropriate—it's not telling it like it is. And these mis-cues are often experienced as pain. If the disturbance is great enough, it will upset the blood supply to an area such as the hand so badly as to result in causalgia, a disease in which the blood supply is seriously diminished. Cases of such severity are rare, but lesser degrees of such disturbances occur fairly often.

Moreover, the autonomic nervous system tends to work in body segments, seldom influencing, say, only the thumb. It ordinarily works for the whole arm, and it may include the arm, upper chest, and head, or the leg and half the body—that's another regional autonomic area. Through another little switch, it may include the lower half of the body. There are variations from person to person, but most symptoms representing dysfunctions of the autonomic nervous system occur in people who are physically ill, especially when there is chronic pain, or when there has been a lot of surgery or physical trauma to the body. The more serious the disease and the longer the illness continues, the greater the chance of additional problems in other organs under the influence of continuing stress.

By purposefully achieving self-regulation of the autonomic nervous system, the dysfunction and pain can be overcome. The nervous system is very flexible; it is not at all a fixed, static thing. Nerve pathways can be changed. Functions of cells can change or be changed, and if the alteration in function goes on long enough, a totally new pattern is set up. In the instance of a tumor, the brain can learn to order the arteries that nourish the tissue to contract and in doing so deprive the tumor of its nourishment and allow it to be reabsorbed and to disappear. What you want to do is program your nervous system to set up good patterns, pleasant patterns. This is what we are teaching in this book.

If we cut the nerve that supplies the biceps muscle —the one that bends your arm up—and we cut the nerve from the triceps muscle—it does the straightening of the arm—and we sew these two nerves crosswise so that the triceps nerve comes into the biceps muscle and the biceps nerve goes into the triceps muscle, we alter the information coming in on that nerve as well as the information going out. The nerve cell in the spinal cord gets new information: The stimulation of the triceps nerve is actually coming from the biceps muscle, and vice versa.

After this alteration of activity has gone on for only six months, if we were to put an electrode into the nerve cell and record from it electrically, it will have changed its functions by 50 percent so that the biceps nerve cell looks like a crazy mixture of triceps and biceps, and it will have picked up from somewhere, presumably by sprouting or by opening up pathways that are there but not normally seen, connections from the group of muscles that worked with the triceps, so the biceps nerve cell will no longer look like a biceps nerve cell. It will have part of the biceps field and part of the triceps field. The same thing occurs with the triceps nerve cell.

Now all that took place just because there was an artificial physical interchange between the two nerves, because of a physical alteration of the nerve function. It's not a very practical way and it doesn't have much use, but as an experiment it demonstrates that such changes are possible.

As you read further, remember that 85 percent of all symptoms represent a reaction to emotional stress. And *every* illness, whatever the interrelating of other factors, is influenced strongly by emotional stress or calm. Often the outcome, recovery or continuing disability, will hinge upon positive thinking and willpower. Systematic practice of Biogenics allows control of 80 percent of symptoms and represents the best-known program for the maintenance of health. You then become increasingly competent in managing responsibilities, obligations, and opportunities, and in resolving conflicts of the past. However, will power and positive thinking are not necessarily enough. Perfect balance between will and imagination are crucial. What you *believe,* even subconsciously, will ultimately prevail.

Now look at the accompanying disease chart, which categorizes various health influences according to the amount of control you may exercise over them. As you see, nearly all the factors are self-health related or can be regulated by proper mental training.

Whatever the distress in one's life, an enlightened and integrated mind can resolve the conflict rationally and lovingly. The exact problem is of relatively little concern. What matters is coming to grips with it—accepting those things you cannot alter and rejecting those things you can alter, by changing them.

For instance, I personally don't believe in divorce, which is based on my observations that most people I see who remarry are no happier than they were the first time. Of course there are exceptions, and my view is not important anyway. All I say is, it's your responsibility. If you hate your spouse, if you truly can't stand him or her, you must divorce. And if you don't hate your spouse really, then stop fighting with him or her emotionally. But in any case, come to grips with those things you are upset over, or no divorce will improve your situation. Be sure before you escape from a marriage—or a job—that it's not just your own anxiety and tenseness you are trying to escape.

Consider the case of one woman I knew who kept complaining about her husband and finally exploded. "That so and so. . . . He went out and bought a piano while I have been in the hospital, but refuses to pay my medical bills." If she really feels that way about her husband, why on earth does she remain married to him? His support was practically nil as she was on Medical Assistance anyway!

My advice is, if you can't stand your job, quit it, even if you are sixty years old. Lots of people have begun a totally new and productive career at seventy. I don't believe that anybody at any age is incapable of finding a new job. It may be harder for some, depending upon one's education and the current economic scene, but it depends to a much greater extent upon what one is willing to do. You and only you can look within yourself and know what it is that ties you up in knots. Individuals have to learn to talk with themselves,

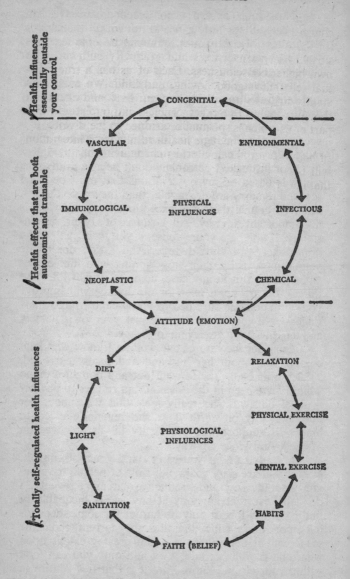

Health influences essentially outside your control

Health effects that are both autonomic and trainable

Totally self-regulated health influences

CONGENITAL

VASCULAR   ENVIRONMENTAL

IMMUNOLOGICAL   PHYSICAL   INFECTIOUS
                 INFLUENCES

NEOPLASTIC   CHEMICAL

ATTITUDE (EMOTION)

DIET   RELAXATION

                            PHYSICAL EXERCISE

LIGHT   PHYSIOLOGICAL
             INFLUENCES   MENTAL EXERCISE

SANITATION   HABITS

        FAITH (BELIEF)

to face emotional distress, to accept themselves, to change those things they can and not to kill themselves for those things they cannot. You *can* become less sensitive to emotional stress and gradually cultivate your own higher consciousness. Each of us has a true spiritual self that is good, loving, and kind. We must constantly strive to bring love into our lives and direct our thoughts always to our own highest and purest self, that part of us which is spiritual or attuned to the divine.

In the long run, true health results from integration of body, mind, and spirit. In the following chapters, we will begin the exercises designed to help you achieve that integration.

TWO

Beginning Your
Ninety-Day Program

It has been my experience that most people lack faith in their own abilities. What I would like to teach you are certain techniques that don't require your faith in any external event, but that do require mental attention and conscious effort. The techniques do not assume that something is going to come out of the sky, or out of the cosmos, and happen to a passive you; rather they require your active participation in helping your body to be healthy—to tune it up and keep it in tune. And they do require a positive attitude, as well as a faith—in yourself.

Of course, it is not always possible to remake yourself fully, whether your techniques are physical, emotional, or chemical. If you had a leg cut off, I don't believe it is possible to regrow it. If you have a knee that has been surgically fused, so that it is all solid bone with no distinguishable joint, I don't believe any amount of mental control will enable you to open it up. (I think it *is* possible, however, for a good orthopedic surgeon to put in a whole new knee joint.) The power of our mental techniques, then, is clearly limited to physically reversible processes. So what we mean to teach you here is that most of the physical problems that you have are indeed either reversible or controllable. Women with small breasts, for instance, have even been taught with techniques such as these to increase the size of their breasts by as much as 1½ inches. At any rate, you should be able to stop the *advancement* of any disease you are now suffering.

The idea that one could do this mentally, as well as by physical or chemical means, is very old. It certainly goes back to the days of Jesus of Nazareth. He talked about it; He even demonstrated it.

In the East, Tibet and India, for instance, the so-called wise men—the gurus, the swamis, the lamas—have routinely believed in the power of the mind to control the body, even one's very heartbeat. Some of them even claim that they don't have to eat but that like plants they can photosynthesize their food with air, water, and sunlight. Now, I don't know whether they can do that—to my knowledge, it hasn't really been tested. But scientific testing of their claims to have control over their heartbeat began about ten years ago. It was found that they did, indeed, have such abilities, that they were capable of instantaneously increasing their heartbeat to 300 pulses per minute. How long they could carry that on is not certain, because the scientists working with them were generally afraid to let them do it for too long; the claim is that they can sustain it for twenty-four hours if they want to. They can also slow their pulse rate to a reasonable level, say, to 40. (Nobody has yet demonstrated that one of them could turn off his heart completely!)

Most of these people who achieve such self-control through various Eastern meditation techniques also have instantaneous control over body temperature. The best of them who have been tested can instantaneously raise the temperature of a finger or foot or some part of their body by 8 to 10 degrees. Now, they did not learn to do simply that. Of course, learning to raise the temperature of the thumb wasn't the ultimate goal of their efforts; what they were striving for is what they would call "total self-control."

The concept of teaching people to alter body function through mental effort is becoming increasingly more acceptable, even in the West, and it has been used in this country primarily through the techniques called "biofeedback" by which a person can be taught to change any body process. If, for instance, we wanted you to alter your cortisone level, we would give you a chemical readout of your blood cortisone level and then have you mentally determine that you want to raise it or lower it. When you can *see* the effects of your thinking, you can ultimately learn to effect changes in the function by will.

Interestingly, what has also been discovered is that as you learn control over one body function that you can't ordinarily control, you gain control over a number of other body functions more or less incidentally. The reason is that, just as drugs have various effects other than those for which you take them, a lot of your body functions are interrelated, too. When you learn to balance some part of your automatically functioning activities, many other autonomic or automatic activities are affected at the same time, often resulting in normalization. Also, a more generalized self-regulation, such as increasing one's blood circulation to the hand, can have a specific effect, such as relieving a migraine headache.

The purpose of this book is to teach you the ways we have now of reducing the ill effects of distress upon various body functions, and I cannot overemphasize the significance of such effects. The thousands of automatic functions (heartbeat, digestion, kidney functions, hormone and enzyme production, to mention a few), which are coordinated by the autonomic nervous system, are all regulated by the hypothalamus, the master switch in the brain, *which is completely surrounded by that part of the brain that manages emotions.* So it's easy to understand what an endless variety of influences emotional stress has throughout the body.

For example, the most prominent reaction to emotional stress is an increased output of adrenalin and cortisone. Although both hormones are essential to life, in excess they race the body's functions and tend to wear it out. Blood pressure is elevated; the heart beats harder and more rapidly; blood salts are altered; kidneys are forced to work harder; the stomach produces more acidity and the entire intestinal tract may move sluggishly (or, alternatively, more rapidly and with irritation); circulation of blood in the skin is decreased; sweating increases; salivation is influenced; resistance to infections or cancer is reduced; susceptibility to allergies increases; and so on and on.

Biogenics, as used in this book, consists in mental exercises or programs designed to help you stabilize the autonomic nervous system. Once you achieve such control, emotional stress is regularly canceled, and no longer harmful to the body. And each day you will tune in, more and more to the universal life force—you may want to call it God—which works with your highest inner being to achieve physical, mental, and spiritual health.

If you intend to follow the program as developed in this book, you must plan on doing a certain amount of practicing. Just as virtuosity on the violin requires many hours of practice, perfecting the techniques of Biogenics takes practice, too. And the greater the damage that's been done, the greater the time and effort required to repair it. Most people, practicing 45 minutes a day (divided up into three 15-minute sessions) for six to ten months, are able to achieve excellent self-regulation of the autonomic nervous system. The exercises in this book are designed to fit into such a practice routine.

Since stress builds tension, both physical and emotional, Biogenics begins with relaxation, and your ability to relax may eventually be the determining factor in preventing disease or death. Actually, I began learning Biogenics exercises to find techniques for helping my chronic-pain patients. After six months of teaching these, I realized they were so good that I used this system to help overcome my own chronic neck problem which had persisted despite two "disc" operations. At the same time, I learned to be much more relaxed most of the time, and it's amazing how much energy one saves by regular relaxing!

There are dozens of techniques for relaxation. Relaxation—while remaining awake—is a delightfully pleasant experience worth cultivating. Many people are so tense they never relax except during sleep; how much they miss of the joys of life!

Once you've relaxed, you will learn to go within your own mind, to examine yourself objectively without outside influences, and in this state you learn to savor each moment without concern for any other, to *be, as of now.* And in this state of internal awareness you can program the physiology of your body by repeating the appropriate suggestions to it and by visualizing the desired goals. Once you learn the techniques this book will be teaching you, you will become so acutely aware of the functions of your body that you will know where stress is affecting you and you'll be able to avoid such wasteful wear and tear. The entire process makes you feel better. And you'll begin to appreciate how nice it is to feel good. It is both pleasant and desirable that you actually *feel good.* So relax and enjoy it.

The first step in relaxing is to find a comfortable position. For most people this means lying flat on your back with hands and legs uncrossed. If you're sitting, you should have your back as straight as possible, legs and hands uncrossed and in a restful position. Eventually you'll learn to relax in any position, but at first it's easiest to relax flat on your back.

Your next goal is to achieve a fixed concentration —to focus your attention upon a specific mental activity so that distracting thoughts and emotions don't interfere. I realize that you won't relax perfectly just by being told to relax, but it isn't so difficult if you begin by telling *yourself* to RELAX. And stop thinking about anything else. Always begin by closing your eyes and taking a deep breath—enjoy the pleasure of feeling yourself breathe.

If you're serious about improving your health, now's the time to begin! Read the exercise and then do it.

Day 1

Assume your posture, close your eyes, and breathe slowly in and out. As you breathe in, say quietly to yourself, "I am" as you breathe out, say to yourself, "relaxed."

To start, you may count on your fingers 40 *deep, slow* breaths. This will take about 10 minutes. Soon you will learn to judge for yourself how long 10 minutes is and to stop at the proper time. Remember, stay awake, and enjoy the experience.

End by taking a deep breath, opening your eyes, and stretching comfortably to feel all the parts of your body reawakening. Relaxation is in reality a technique for deep body rest or sleep while the mind remains conscious.

The second time you practice today, say to yourself and do what you say:

I visualize the number "3." I take a deep breath, continuing to visualize "3," and I repeat 3–3–3 as I breathe out.

I visualize the number "2." I take another deep, pleasant breath, and as I breathe out, I repeat 2–2–2.

I visualize the number "1." I take a deep, pleasant breath, and as I breathe out, I repeat 1–1–1.

I feel myself relaxing deeper and deeper. I deepen the relaxation by visualizing myself stepping onto the top of an escalator, and I breathe deeply and slowly in and out. And as I see myself descending on the escalator, into a deeper and deeper state of relaxation, I count 10–9–8–7–6–5–4–3–2–1.

I am now deeply and pleasantly relaxed.

Now take a deep breath, open your eyes, and stretch to reawaken all the parts of your body.

The third time you practice today, proceed this way:

Relax, close your eyes. Then as you breathe in, imagine you are breathing in through your feet, and as you breathe out, imagine that your breath is washing out and cleansing your feet. (Repeat 10 breaths.) Then do the same for your

Legs	Arms
Pelvis	Neck
Abdomen	Head
Back	Body as a whole
Chest	

This particular exercise is one of the most important in this book. If you have free time during the day, spend a few minutes breathing this way, inhaling through your body as a whole and cleansing your body as you breathe out through your entire body. The concept may be somewhat difficult to grasp at first; just accept it as an exercise in imagination.

To apply the exercise to a specific pain or disease in some part of your body, sit in a relaxed way, preferably in the fresh air or near a source of fresh air and breathe in and out through that part of your body for 10 to 30 minutes. Always complete the exercise by breathing through the body as a whole for at least 10 breaths.

Practice this technique many times daily, whenever you have a few moments. The more you practice, the more you'll benefit. Only through repetition can changes be effected in the autonomic nervous system. Repetition of Biogenics exercises is the most important factor in success. Only with constant repetition can you "get through" to your subconscious mind and the central management system, the hypothalamus and the limbic system. It seems essential that habits be patterned and programmed repeatedly into the lower levels of consciousness in order to obtain good effects.

There is nothing to be gained by screaming and yelling and wailing and gnashing your teeth and saying, "It hasn't worked yet." The more you let yourself feel that way, the less likely it is that the technique will be effective. Biogenics won't work overnight. If it did, there would be no need for doing the exercises, because you could learn things so easily and it would become a part of you so quickly that you wouldn't need the kind of reinforcement we are talking about.

Also, if you find yourself shifting around constantly during the exercises, you know you aren't practicing. You can't be. Learning to focus your attention isn't easy and I never said it was. The real question is, is your health worth 45 minutes a day? If you agree it is, resolve to set aside several periods of time each day to work on it. It's really as important as eating for your personality needs the nourishment of love and care, as much as your body needs food.

Now, let's look at the development of Biogenics historically.

THREE

Biogenics®-Its History and What It Has to Offer

Although the use of positive mental programming to overcome stress is as old as the practice of medicine itself, it has only become widespread and achieved a genuine scientific basis in this century.

Emil Coué, a pharmacist from Troyes, France, born in 1857, became very much interested in the healing power of the mind. In 1910 he opened a free clinic at Nancy, which he ran for many years. Finally in 1922, only four years before his death, he published his first widely distributed work.

He considered what he was doing to be essentially suggestion, or auto-suggestion; sometimes he called it "conscious auto-suggestion." One of the basic tenets of his work was that the will always yields to the imagination. (It is worth remembering that early in this century the autonomic nervous system was called "the imaginative nervous system.") His favorite statement was, "in the conflict between the will and the imagination, the force of the imagination is in direct ratio to the square of the will,"* that is, the power of the imagination is

---

*Emil Coué and C. H. Brooks: *Suggestion and Auto-suggestion,* New York, Samuel Weister, 1974, a reprint of "Self Mastery through Conscious Auto-suggestion" by Emil Coué and "The Practice of Auto-suggestion by the Method of Emil Coué" by C. H. Brooks.

far greater than that of the will. Accordingly, he felt it a gross error to advise people to train their will when they really should be training their imagination—their most important faculty: "It is an absolute rule that admits of no exception . . . we only cease to be puppets when we have learned to guide our imagination." He contended that if a person persuades himself through his imagination that he can do a certain thing—provided it is physically possible—then he will, in fact, be able to do it no matter how difficult it may be. And, by the same token, if a person imagines that the simplest task in the world is beyond his abilities, then "molehills become for [him] unscalable mountains." Thus, we are what we think we are, and the fear of failure becomes in itself the cause for failure.

In beginning his work with patients, Coué used some of the standard hypnotic techniques. For instance, he would have the subject clasp his hands in front of himself until his fingers trembled. Keeping his own hand on the patient, he would then look the subject straight in the eye and ask him to squeeze his hands together even more tightly, telling him repeatedly that he could not unclasp his fingers. He would then say, "I am going to count to three and when I reach the number three, you will be unable to separate your hands." The patient was instructed to think all the while, "I cannot do it, I cannot do it," and, of course, would then find it impossible to separate his hands. If the patient was concentrating properly, his fingers not only would remain clasped but would become even more tightly clasped. Then the patient would be asked to say, "I can do it," and his fingers would separate.

Coué emphasized that if the patient's fingers did not lock, he had not been properly thinking, "I cannot do it." Patients who did not obtain satisfactory results with auto-suggestion failed either because they lacked confidence or because they tried too hard and did not allow their bodies to respond to their imagination. To make good suggestions, Coué pointed out, it was necessary to do it *without effort,* since effort implies the use of will or willpower, which should be put aside entirely in auto-suggestion. This point, we were to learn years later in autogenic therapy, was well founded.

Because, according to Coué, "every one of our thoughts, good or bad, becomes concrete, materializes and becomes, in short, a reality," people who predict they will have a headache on a certain day or because of a certain event will, indeed, be suffering from that headache when such a time comes around. He emphasized that one should always be careful about speaking of illnesses in front of children, who are particularly susceptible to auto-suggestion, and should only be exposed to the idea that good health is the normal state for man and sickness is abnormal, a "sort of back-sliding which may be avoided by living in a temperate, regular way." He believed that children should be encouraged to regard work and study as pleasant activities, for "all we think becomes true for us." He emphasized to his patients that whenever gloomy thoughts came to them, they should quietly transfer their attention to something brighter. He felt that happiness could thus be wooed and won, since it was more native to the human mind than negative preoccupations.

Since "every thought entirely filling our mind becomes true for us and tends to transform itself into action," an organic disease could become more severe by allowing the mind to dwell upon it and, in so doing, directing, "our life force to our own destruction." Anyone who listens to numerous suggestions that he is ill has gone a long way toward actually becoming ill. And on the same premise, supplanting such gloomy thoughts with *curative* auto-suggestion would effect healing. In this way, Coué felt, it would be possible in many cases for patients to stop hemorrhages, relieve constipation, shrink fibrous tumors, and cure paralysis, tuberculosis, varicose ulcers, and other diseases. He felt that if the unconscious—the imagination—accepted the idea of dispensing with such diseases and their symptoms, they would indeed disappear. He believed that except for the mentally undeveloped who are unable to understand what is said to them and those who are *unwilling* to understand, any patient is capable of responding to auto-suggestion/The cure of chronic disease could then be effected in about six months.

According to his methods, conditions for treatment were perfect as long as will and thought and imagination were in harmony. That concept is the basis for the famous phrase he encouraged his patients to repeat twenty times to themselves upon waking, mechanically moving their lips:/Every day in every way I am getting better and better." He felt that the desire and the statement had to be expressed without passion and without will/but with absolute confidence. He also found effective such general phrases as/"I am going to be cured," or in the case of physical pain, "it is going away," or "it is going."/He also had specific suggestions for specific diseases/For asthma, for instance, there was—

> *From this day forward, my breathing will become rapidly easier. My organism will do all that is necessary to restore perfect health to my lungs /and bronchial passages. I shall be able to undergo any exertion without inconvenience. My breathing will be free, deep, and delightful. I shall sleep calmly and peacefully with a maximum refreshment and repose, and I will awake cheerful and look forward with pleasure to the day's task.**

/He encouraged his patients as they got into bed at night to assume a comfortable position, practice general relaxation of all the muscles of their bodies, and close their eyes/As they drifted into the "stage of semiconsciousness akin to that of daydreaming," it would be possible to introduce into the mind any desired idea. /The unconscious mind would then turn thought into reality—would make the wish come true, so to speak. (Such concepts are very similar to some of the advanced organ-specific phrases of present-day autogenic therapy, as we will see later in the 90-day program.) One of Coué's most startling statements at the time was that/'contrary to common opinion, physical dis-

---

*Ibid., pages 139–140.

eases are generally far more easily cured than mental ones."

The publication in 1929 of Edmond Jacobson's *Progressive Relaxation* became another landmark in psychophysiological medicine. Jacobson, a Chicago physician, expressed ideas very different from those of Coué, his emphasis being on teaching people to relax, which, he contended, required neither imagination, will-power, nor self- nor auto-suggestion. His work was based on the tenet that just as all thought processes diminish during extreme musclar relaxation, so do emotions. He believed that muscular elements appear in all emotions and relaxation is the opposite of emotion: "The subjective experience of emotion is largely derived from intense proprioceptive impulses"—those arising from within oneself. Hence, since the hypothalamus and deep brain structures are put into a state of relaxation when visual and auditory imagery cease, the quieting of emotions would be the natural outcome of deep muscular relaxation.

According to Jacobson, whether or not the mind became blank was unimportant. But even though he put no emphasis on mental exercise or formal suggestion, he found, interestingly, that "the cerebral activity of attention apparently diminished in the presence of advancing relaxation" and that in brief periods of absolutely perfect relaxation, all imagery—visual, auditory, and so on—is totally absent.

Contrary to the theories we'll discuss later in autogenic training and those prominent in Emil Coué's work, he emphasized that visual or auditory imagery, either spontaneous or suggested from an outside source, is always accompanied by sensations of tension. He contended that his patients who were highly skilled in relaxation all agreed that visual imagery always provokes tension, in the ocular muscles, at least, and that without that slight tension the images will not appear.

His methods began by having the patient lie comfortably on his back with his arms at his sides and his legs uncrossed. The sitting position could also be used.

Although he treated as many as eight patients at a time, he always had them in different rooms and would walk from room to room as he supervised their practicing of the muscle tension followed by relaxation.

Jacobson believed that if he taught patients to recognize the contractions of muscles, they would notice the opposite—the relaxation of those muscles. To show the patients "what not to do," he had them practice tensing various muscles, following a specific order throughout the body. The purpose of these muscle-tensing exercises was to point out that relaxation requires no effort whereas contraction does. He always had the patients work with only one muscle group at a time, and he always emphasized that the patient should not *observe* what is happening but only *feel* it. Patients were to practice 5 to 15 minutes a day and to devote their entire first period of practice to, for instance, just the biceps group, or to several muscle groups, and then let those muscles become limp. The patient would then learn quickly to go through the entire body, first tensing and then relaxing.

Included in Jacobson's work was the measuring of a variety of physiological activities during deep muscle relaxation, including gastric secretions and galvanic skin response, or GSR. The latter, he discovered, is a useful gauge of the degree of relaxation being experienced. It measures the resistance of the skin to passage of minute quantities of electricity, such that the more relaxed one is, the *higher* the resistance, the less relaxed, the lower one's resistance. Thus, a tense individual is *more* susceptible to passage of electricity.

He noted excellent clinical results in treating a rather large number of diseases, including mucous colitis, spastic esophagus (globus hystericus), chronic insomnia, compulsion neurosis, mild phobias, neurasthenia, easy fatigability, anxiety neurosis, cardiac neurosis, compulsive tic, depression, Graves' disease (hyperthyroidism), hypochondria, generalized spastic paresis, and stuttering and stammering.

Again it appears that simple, deep muscle relaxation, even without programmed mental activity or psychophysiological programming, can lead to significant improvement in autonomic nervous system function and control of many of the psychosomatic or psychophysiological illnesses.

The year 1932 saw the publication of the definitive work in the field of autogenic training—that of J. H. Schultz,* who was later joined by Wolfgang Luthe. Dr. Schultz, a German psychiatrist and a contemporary of Freud, does not give any particular credit to possible influences of either Coué or Jacobson, but, rather, related autogenic techniques primarily to earlier studies in hypnosis. To Schultz, autogenic therapy consisted in what he called "mental manipulation" of body functions, and he, like so many others before and after, felt that the ultimate changes evolving from such practice occurred in the diencephalon, that portion of the brain containing the hypothalamus.

Schultz emphasized that autogenics is a *specific state*, which leads to self-normalization or self-regulation, and that it works in exact opposition to the physiological alterations induced by stress. The shift into this "autogenic state," he maintained, is encouraged by conditions that reduce sensations, and regular, if brief, sessions of passive concentration on psychophysiologically adapted stimuli (those autogenic formulae designed to balance body functions) would gradually balance the physiology or the autonomic nervous system of the body.

It was Schultz and Luthe, in fact, who devised the six exercises that became the standard ones used in present-day autogenic techniques for stabilization, or auto-regulation, of circulation, respiration, and neuromuscular activity. The phrases that form the basis of the six exercises are:

My arms and legs are heavy.

My arms and legs are warm.

My heartbeat is calm and regular.

*J. H. Schultz, *Das Autogene Training*, George Thieme Verlag, Stuttgart, 1932.

It breathes me.

My abdomen is warm.

My forehead is cool.

With satisfactory practice of autogenic exercises, patients wind up in a "neutral autogenic state" or one of "increased vigilance." In such a state, patients reportedly have a markedly increased awareness of internal stimuli and decreased discrimination among and reactivity to external stimuli. During the above mental exercises, the skeletal muscles begin to relax just from the patient's concentration on feelings of heaviness. Interestingly, the knee jerk reflex is diminished or even absent during autogenic therapy—which, incidentally, was also the case with Jacobson's technique whereby the patients arrived at relaxation by tensing the muscles first and then relaxing without any mental focusing.

Further, people who have become accomplished at autogenic exercise develop an increased resistance of galvanic skin response, showing up on the graph as a smoother curve in response to stimulation. Such a response is in contrast to the rather erratic and volatile curve of patients who have not been so indoctrinated— evidence that the trained patients are more relaxed. An interesting case showing the connection of GSR with stress is that of one of my patients who controlled her pain with a simple electrical stimulator (to be mentioned later). When the woman's son was arrested, thus increasing her stress, her skin burned at levels previously well tolerated. The physiological improvement with autogenics is similar to that obtained in deep muscle relaxation; similar results have also been noted in Transcendental Meditation.

It takes most patients from three to six months to go through the six phrases in the standard autogenic training technique. However, by that stage, a patient is able with 20 or 30 *seconds* of concentration on the six phrases to feel as if his or her body were warm and heavy, a resting mass. I think it is important to have the patient develop the sensation that his body is totally numb or even absent, as if his mind were floating up above his body, which is lying totally numb below, or even that the body is asleep and the mind awake. I have found that almost any patient sleeps better within a few days of beginning the intense Biogenic approach we use even for those who require special help, phrases such as "I am relaxing deeper and deeper," or "I am progressing deeper toward normal, relaxing sleep," certainly seem effective.

It should be noted that sudden interruption of the autogenic exercises is quite undesirable. It is best to practice where one is undisturbed and where the atmosphere is tranquil. As you improve with practice you will be able to induce your state of relaxation in almost any environment, but try whenever possible to practice without interference—including that of drugs. Barbiturates interfere negatively with the balancing process of autogenic training, although small doses of certain tranquilizers may help patients who are significantly distressed. In general, however, it is best to avoid drugs. *Do not,* of course, *stop* taking any drug without your physician's advice.

Regarding specific diseases, clinical therapeutic experience with autogenic training has been achieved in a great variety of illnesses. Although autogenic training will not alter the underlying pathology of such central nervous system diseases as Parkinsonism, multiple sclerosis, and Huntington's chorea, it can help the patients cope with associated or superimposed functional disorders, such as the emotional excitement and fatigue which aggravate tremor and the cramp and pain in the back of the leg in Parkinsonism, and even muscular rigidity. A small number of patients have experienced a gradual reduction in both tremor and rigidity as the anxiety and emotional excesses become normalized. There have even been occasional clinical impressions that regular autogenic practice decreases the frequency of exacerbations and the downhill course in multiple sclerosis.

On the other hand, results have been consistently excellent in the use of autogenics in treating functional tremors such as benign, essential, and other tremors as-

sociated with chronic and acute anxiety. Many forms
of muscular tics, such as blepharospasms (jerky eyelids) and spasmotic torticollis (a twisted neck) have
been known to respond to autogenic training. Torticollis
is even more significantly improved when EMG (electromyogram—the measurer of muscle tension biofeedback is included. Satisfactory control of phantom limb
pain and related phenomena has also been reported in
autogenic training, and narcolepsy has been improved
in five reported cases with three of the cases being
cured.

In most cases of severe mental deterioration or
brain damage, no significant benefit has been reported.
Occasionally, however, even in a severely damaged patient some of the emotional debility can be improved
with a great deal of specialized work. Patients with
various types of brain injury have been reported to
sleep better, to feel more emotionally secure and stable,
to be more efficient at their jobs, to have an improved
social life and a more open life style, and to have been
able to give up smoking or drinking.

It is not surprising that numerous authors have reported that regular practice of autogenic standard exercises improves the course of epilepsy with 50 to 75
percent of the patients having been noted as having
fewer and milder seizures. EEG (electroencephalogram
—brain wave tracings) biofeedback probably will have
the same effect. Even when there is no improvement in
the number or intensity of the seizures, desirable personality and behavioral changes have been noted, with
patients tending, say, to become less irritable or less
aggressive.

Even though conversion hysteria and severe, ob-
sessive compulsion reactions in severely accident-prone
patients are difficult to treat, depression, phobias, and
anxiety are likely to respond to autogenic training. At
least 75 percent of patients with various types of neu-
roses and psychoneuroses respond well to autogenic
training. People with more serious mental problems
such as psychotic depression or severe melancholia may
improve very significantly after extensive practice of
autogenic training, especially in group training. In many

cases of the severely depressed, the patient often makes no progress at all for several weeks, then breaks down with a crying catharsis, and, after more work, eventually achieves much greater emotional stability. Sexual psychopaths also have been noted to benefit from autogenic therapy if given general psychotherapeutic support.

Although schizophrenia and other more serious psychotic disorders have been treated successfully with autogenic therapy, such patients require the very close supervision of psychiatrists and should not undertake training in autogenic courses outside a psychiatrist's office without his referral. What has been known to happen in courses such as the mind-control classes, which are widely offered to the general public in this country, is that many patients who are borderline psychotics break down and require institutionalization after taking those courses. Patients who are severely paranoid also may become worse during autogenic therapy as they believe that someone else is trying to take control of them; thus psychotics should practice autogenics only under psychiatric care!

The balancing of the autonomic functions is also significant help in treating drug addicts and alcoholics. Addictions to narcotics, to nicotine or smoking, and to alcohol have all been very successfully treated with autogenic therapy. Again, the patients do better in group sessions where they may have more significant support during the training process. (The greatest difficulty in treating alcoholism, of course, is motivating the patient to want to stop drinking. In one study, only 44 percent of the alcoholic patients continued the training after the first four sessions. I wonder whether the lack of persistence wouldn't be due primarily to the tedious, monotonous way in which the heaviness formula is introduced. Schultz took up to six weeks just having patients repeat "My right hand is heavy." I believe that if more emotionally stimulating and varied exercises were used, one might be able to secure the continuing participation of a greater percentage of alcoholics.)

The greatest successes with autogenic training and

the really outstanding cases have been in the most common psychosomatic or psychophysiological disturbances: constipation, colitis, gastritis, peptic ulcer, spastic colon, many functional disorders of the gallbladder and bioducts, loss of appetite, nausea and vomiting, and hemorrhoids. In 80 percent of the cases, patients with difficulties in sexual performance, headaches, various respiratory complaints, gastrointestinal and cardiac complaints, phobias, poor emotional stability, muscular tension and spasms, anxiety, and insomnia are noted to improve over a six- to ten-week period.

During the early practice of autogenic training, there is often an increase in intestinal activity with rumbling and splashing sounds, which are presumably a reaction to the autonomic regulation beginning to take place and indicative of the generalized response of the autonomic nervous system.

Regular practice of autogenic exercises has been greatly beneficial to patients who are overweight, as it reduces anxiety and tension as well as their weight. Many undesirable habits, such as stammering, nail biting, eating or chewing on hair, and bed-wetting, seem to be reactions to stress, and so autogenics once again has been found to be most helpful.

Autogenic training has been used by athletes as well as by various creative artists. Favorable effects of its use have been reported in a variety of amateur sports ranging from golf to hockey and including baseball, tennis, judo, skiing, and cycling. Better performance, increased coordination, greater endurance, and faster recuperation from injury have all been reported. Autogenic training has also been found to be extremely useful by a number of Olympic champions. Some work has also been done with professional sportsmen.

I have read a program called psychogenics, which claims to be a means of building up tremendous physical power and size. It uses the first two of the basic Schultz phrases, "My arm is heavy" and "My arm is warm," in a focused mental exercise in combination with physical exercise. There are no published statistics to corroborate statements made in the course, but, for whatever it is worth, this method is reported to work far better than exercise alone.

Significant improvement in creativity and productivity, decreased fatigue, greater feelings of happiness, and improved sleep have all been reported in businessmen who have undertaken regular autogenic training. In Germany, a number of autogenic training sessions have been carried out under the auspices of various business organizations, such as the chambers of commerce, to help the personnel of large companies, railroads, and telephone service centers. Increased health and efficiency, decreased absenteeism, fewer errors and accidents, improved interpersonal relationships, and overall lessening of stress have been reported. In those situations dealing with relatively normal individuals, the training has usually been done in sessions of one and a half hours once a week for five weeks and then every two weeks for six weeks. Each hour-and-a-half session is devoted to discussion of training difficulties, and discussion and instruction of the next standard formula (of the six mentioned earlier).

In groups, training works better when members have similar social and cultural backgrounds. It has also been found that it's best if the therapist is not an employee of the organization whenever businesses use autogenic training.

Autogenics has also been used by the Russian astronauts. It has been reported to be of great help as well in stressful situations such as the case of a physician who crossed the Atlantic in a one-man, kayak-type boat. All such evidence seems to suggest that autogenics is particularly useful to people who are in any kind of hazardous situation or under physical or emotional strain.

It has been noted that patients who are very well trained in autogenics can lower their pulse rate by 25 percent and even those who are just short-term practitioners can lower it about 10 percent. Similar changes, incidentally, have also been noted in Zen training and in yoga, as well as Transcendental Meditation, behavioral therapy, and other forms of therapy, and even during altered states of consciousness brought about by drugs. I find no proof that the autogenic state is significantly different from some of these other physiologically altered states of consciousness. Obviously if unpleasant symptoms develop during the exercises, then you should either terminate the exercises or alter the particular psychophysiological exercises you are doing.

Unfortunately, very little has been written for the public about the field of autogenic training. Of some 2,500 publications related to such subjects as autogenic therapy, self-hypnosis, and so on, fewer than 10 percent are in English, and most of the others are in Japanese or foreign publications that have no significant circulation in the American medical press.

Actually, it was the introduction of biofeedback that made the whole field of autogenic training even as available as it is in the United States, which isn't very available at all. Biofeedback is a therapeutic device that helps a patient learn to modify and balance certain physiological functions and states of mind previously believed not subject to voluntary regulation by feeding back to the patient the results of his mental exercises. Essentially, biofeedback is the reporting to the patient of changes in the body brought about by thinking. When one thinks "my right hand is warm" it actually becomes warm.

There are various types of biofeedback training, including brain wave training, in which the patient learns to modify his brain wave output; temperature biofeedback training, in which one learns to raise or lower the skin temperature of a portion of the body; and EMG (electromyogram) training, in which one learns to relax certain muscles more effectively. Many other types of biofeedback training are being developed or proposed for self-regulation of almost any physiological activity. (I personally have the most clinical experience with temperature regulation and GSR biofeedback.)

In biofeedback training, the patient is supplied with a device that picks up tiny variations in a particular body function. These changes are immediately relayed back to the patient in the form of visual or auditory feedback signals so that he can detect minute variations in the selected function and attempt to make desired changes. Over a period of days (or sometimes weeks) he uses the biofeedback machine for about 30 minutes a day and follows simple instructions which help him to *begin* to modify and, later, to balance that particular function by watching the variations in his device.

The biofeedback machines are battery-driven electronic devices calibrated to pick up extremely small electrical or temperature changes as they take place. These minute changes (often as tiny as one millionth of a volt) are converted to signals a subject can recognize, which allows him to know immediately when changes occur. The machine itself does not exert any form of control over the patient's functions—it only tells him what the body is doing.

Once a patient knows what is going on inside his body, he can begin to associate those changes in his body functions with subtle changes in his conscious feelings—his subjective awareness. He may notice feelings of warmth, of contentment or solitude, of relaxation, and so on, which occur when the biofeedback device tells him that he is producing the desirable change in the function being monitored. With continued practice, the patient often finds, over a period of days or weeks, that his appreciation of his subjective feelings is enhanced; eventually he is able to anticipate the biofeedback signals and has to depend less and less on the machine to know when, for example, he is producing the desired brain waves or is changing the temperature of a part of his body.

At that point when he has learned to use his own awareness to tell him about his internal functions and no longer needs an external device to feed signals back to him, the patient has learned to consciously exert control over a previously uncontrollable function of his body—a function that had been there all the time but which he had never learned to use. But the patient should not stop at that point. Just as one's vocal talents are not developed as soon as one learns to say "da-da" or "water," the patient should continue to develop his new talent.

The possibilities of what biofeedback has to offer are endless. Some people find it difficult, say, to relax, or to stop feeling worried, tense, or frustrated about some aspect of their lives. The techniques learned in biofeedback training may provide them with an alternative to psychiatric treatment or tranquilizers or alcohol —one that is more acceptable, more rational; and most important, allows them to rebalance their *own* functioning, without having to depend on someone else or on drugs. In other words, they can learn to tell their bodies and their minds what to do, instead of their bodies and minds telling them what to do. They can become the captain of their own ship. In the long run, they no longer have to take some drug or to talk out their problems with someone else, and they can save considerable money and time, not to mention receiving the benefits of enhanced self-confidence and independence.

To the best of our knowledge, biofeedback has no real adverse side effects, which *all* drugs potentially have. Then, you say, why isn't it being more widely used? There are a number of reasons. First, it is new, just emerging from the laboratory, and consequently it has not been in use with patients on any large scale. Second, the machines needed in training have been, and to some degree, still are, prohibitively expensive—individual doctors and patients simply cannot afford them. Third, our society has taught us to expect immediate and lasting relief from a pill, an operation, or a variety of other forms of therapy so that we lack the patience for such a slow process. Finally, attitudes in medicine change too slowly for a new approach to be widely accepted, particularly when the effects of a new kind of therapy are not always immediate.

Nevertheless, biofeedback has been shown to be of great value in treating certain chronic conditions, and will be broadened to include others in the near future. It holds great promise, and it appears free of the risks, inherent to other therapies, of making problems worse or creating new ones.

In addition, biofeedback places on the patients' shoulders the primary responsibility for "getting well." The major emphasis is on teaching him to help himself —both physically and mentally, because change in one without change in the other is usually ineffective and short-lived. He is capable of learning a variety of techniques that can allow him to take charge of himself to a greater degree.

However, biofeedback, to be effective, must be applied in conjunction with mental exercises. And since exercises in which one tunes in to sensations from the body are actually sensory biofeedback, it appears that the term Biogenics is a more appropriate one to apply to the whole concept of biofeedback and autogenic training, both of which are really the basis of a healthy, well-balanced life.

(I should like to emphasize that none of the complicated, expensive machines normally used in biofeedback are needed to accomplish self-regulation. The entire program can be quite adequately carried on by practicing the Biogenics exercises taught in this book. If you need proof that your body is responding, you can work with a small thermometer as will be explained later.)

In discussing Biogenics, what we are really talking about is *body-mind harmony,* not control over the mind. You've got control over your mind whenever you want to exercise that control. That is simply a question of desire. But balancing the body is something you work at through your mind and in order to achieve that balance you have to program yourself and your mind regularly.

Of course, many other techniques purporting to be methods for achieving something like body-mind harmony stand in varying degrees of good—and ill—favor today. Three such systems are autogenics, hypnosis, and Transcendental Meditation. It should be noted, however, that all three, like Biogenics, begin with relaxation, and *there the similarity ends.* In hypnosis, one suppresses his consciousness while passively accepting suggestions. In TM there is an unusual amount of gobbledygook and concentration upon a meaningless mantra, the object being to attain a passive state of nothingness. But turning off your mind is not, in my judgment, a worthy goal. Your mind, after all, is the agency through which insight, wisdom and illumination come to you. Passivity is not a desirable trait; meaningful and considered insight *is*.

In Biogenics your body is relaxed and physiologically balanced; your mind is poised, *alert,* at peace. If while in a Biogenic state you place yourself in touch with your own higher spiritual self, the God force within you, then you can reflect upon and analyze your problems and integrate them into a more harmonious life. You can seek and purposefully choose the healthiest, most loving path. By acknowledging—and forgiving—your own faults and recognizing—and capitalizing on—your own strengths, you can integrate and balance yourself until only a healthy life force exists within.

After discussing what Biogenics offers, a comment on what it doesn't offer is appropriate. For, although with proper and thorough application Biogenics can relieve most symptoms it is *not* an alternative to conventional medicine. And, of course, many disorders and diseases will surely be fatal unless treated with conventional methods. I would no sooner advise Biogenics for treating a broken bone than I would send you to a witch doctor. He might do a perfectly fine job, mind you (after all they do, sometimes, and not all orthopedists do), but your chances for having the bone heal properly are certainly far better with an orthopedist. If you have a heart attack or develop an infection, you must be taken care of by a medical doctor. Self-regulatory techniques are far too slow when you are seriously ill.

If you have cancer it first ought to be treated with the methods of standard medicine; it might be curable with surgery. When possible, cancer should be treated surgically and with X-ray, and then the residual cells or any tendency for it to regrow can be best handled through Biogenics. *Once medicine has failed to cure a disease, almost any disease, and once you know that there is no specific medical treatment available, then you can afford to use almost any kind of safe mental tech-*

nique. Most people who avoid medicine have a point, but if you are bleeding to death or if you have acute symptoms of almost any sort, you cannot ignore them or start so slow a healing process as Biogenics. They should be taken care of by the best physician available. If there is any question in your mind about a specific medical problem, consult a physician you trust and tell him about all your physical problems. And ask him questions, too. You have a right to know what the risks of any therapy are, if they are known, and if they are not known, you have a right to know that fact, too.

Above all else, maintenance depends upon *you.* It is *your* responsibility. When we say that most symptoms are psychophysiological, we do not imply an abnormal or sick mind. The psychophysiological upset is a normal reaction to the ordinary and extraordinary stresses of everyday life. Sickness develops when those stresses are allowed to persist without physiological rebalancing of the autonomic nervous system and attunement with your highest self.

Health is maintained with regular practicing of good body, mind, and spiritual attunement (Biogenics); adequate physical exercise; and proper nutrition. An adequate amount of sleep (6 to 8 hours daily), relaxation, fun and play, creativity, pleasant work (but not more than 50 hours a week), all blend together to create the best atmosphere for health. Avoidance of harmful habits—smoking, or indulging in excessive alcohol, caffeine, or unneeded drugs—is essential. Uncontrolled worry, anger, depression, guilt, all combine to wear out body and mind much more rapidly than is necessary. Prompt medical attention to new and unusual symptoms is equally necessary to ensure the most rapid recovery possible. Remember, your goal is a healthy balance of will and imagination, desire and belief.

Informed adults have a choice of how they live; it's up to the individual to use the building blocks provided in this book to lay a solid foundation of health.

Remember, Biogenics exercises can enhance *or inhibit* the workings of nature. As you practice, note that Biogenics consists of the following stages:

1. *Relaxation—accomplishing* deep *relaxation within three minutes.*

2. *Being inside self—seeing to it that the mind doesn't wander.*

3. *Being as of now—living in a state of constant awareness of the current moment.*

4. *Attention and attending—focusing one's attention, developing a truly one-track mind, being aware of changes occurring around you.*

5. *Special programming—*
   a. *Word phrases—"organ specific" or goal-oriented exercises to apply to problem symptoms or organs.*
   b. *Visualization—learning to create mental images of the desired improvement.*

Biogenics leads to harmony or balance of body, mind, and spirit. Imbalances are dis-ease. Learn to balance! The daily programs are organized in as simple a way as possible, but to benefit from them, *you must practice.* Reading is fine, but practice achieves the result.

We all have emotions; we all react to them. *But those who cancel the debt regularly do not suffer because of their emotions.* When a patient begins to experience symptoms of stress, he seeks a cause. He and most doctors look for a physical disturbance. Finding one they treat it with drugs or surgery. Not finding one, they blame it on "nerves" and treat the symptom without seeking the cause. If the cause is emotional stress, then the treatment should be aimed at emotional serenity, *peace of mind.* Only when the mind becomes relaxed and peaceful is achieving insight into the cause likely.

Now, let's resume that 90-day program.

FOUR

Relaxation, Relaxation, Relaxation

If you wish to read straight through the book, you may do so directly without experiencing each exercise as you read. Then return to the progressive daily practice sessions. Each day is set up to provide a variety of relaxation. After you complete this chapter you will enjoy choosing your favorite technique or combination of techniques for entering the deepest state of relaxation. First read each day's exercise, then do it. Then, as exercises for the second and third sessions of the day, either repeat the exercise of the day or (and, at any rate, at least once daily) do the third exercise from Day 1—breathing *through* your body (see page 35).*

Day 2

Assume your position. Close your eyes. Take a deep breath and let it out slowly. Then with each *deep, slow* breath in, say to yourself

I am

As you breathe out slowly, say to yourself

---

* If during any practices you develop dizziness, nausea, or any undesirable sensation, terminate the exercise and revert to one you like.

calm and serene

Continue for 10 minutes. Terminate each exercise just as on Day 1, by taking a deep breath, opening your eyes, and stretching comfortably to feel all parts of your body awakening. Remember those three practice sessions each day!

Day 3

Assume position. Close your eyes. Take a deep breath slowly in and out. (These instructions should be followed to begin every exercise.)

As you breath in, say to yourself

I am

At the same time imagine ("see" and "feel") that the electrical energy of your body is circulating over the top of your body from the tips of your toes to the top of your head.

As you breathe out, say to yourself

relaxed

Imagine that the electrical energy of your body is coursing down the back of your body from the top of your head into the soles of your feet.

Repeat for 40 breaths, or 10 minutes, and terminate as usual.

Day 4

As you breathe in, say to yourself

I am

As you breathe out, say to yourself

one

The implication is "at one," or in harmony with life, the universe, and God.

Day 5

As you breathe in, say to yourself

I am

As you breathe out, say

love

Feel the emotion of love as you do your exercise.

Day 6—Energy Balance

The energy-balance technique, used by a number of workers in the field, consists in placing your left hand with the little finger just at the base of the skull in the center of the back of your neck, and your right hand over the upper abdomen with the little finger lying over the navel. Then close your eyes and take 16 deep, slow, complete breaths. This should take approximately 4 minutes. Now reverse your hands, with the right hand on the back of the neck at the base of the skull and the left hand over the upper abdomen with the little finger over the navel. Again, take 16 deep, slow breaths. Finally, place your left hand again on the back of your neck at the base of the skull and place your right hand over the midline in your groin or pubic area and take a final 16 breaths slowly in and out.

Day 7—Talking To Your Body

Begin by systematically thinking of the various parts of your body. Then taking one slow, deep breath with each sentence, say twice for each part

I relax my—	
Scalp	Abdomen
Face	Back
Neck	Pelvis
Shoulders	Hips
Arms	Thighs
Hands	Legs
Chest	Feet

Alternatively, you might say,

My scalp (face, neck, . . .) is relaxing deeper and deeper.

Day 8—Tension To Relaxation

As you repeat each phrase, do it physically. Then relax deeper.

Take in and let out one slow, deep breath with each phrase.

I tense the muscles in my scalp.

Tense them as tight as possible, to the point of trembling.

Now I let go and relax deeper.

Repeat for

Face	**Back**
Neck	**Pelvis**
Shoulders	**Hips**
Arms	**Thighs**
Hands	**Legs**
Chest	**Feet**
Abdomen	

Follow with

I tense my entire body.

then

I let go and relax deeper.

Complete by taking three slow deep breaths before terminating.

Day 9

With each breath, say to yourself 40 times

My right hand is heavy and warm.

If you want to see how beautifully your body is beginning to respond, before you begin, tape the bulb of a small thermometer to the tip of the fleshy part of your right index finger. Wait one minute. Write down the temperature then and the temperature when you finish.

Day 10

With each breath, say to yourself

My heartbeat is calm and regular.

Feel mentally for your heartbeat within your chest.

Day 11

With each breath, say to yourself.

My breathing is relaxed and comfortable.

Day 12

With each breath, say to yourself 40 times

My abdomen is warm.

Feel mentally for deep upper abdomen warmth.

Day 13

With each breath, say to yourself 40 times

My forehead is cool.

Feel mentally for a cool breezy sensation on your forehead.

Day 14

With each breath, say to yourself 40 times

My mind is quiet and still.

Pause a minute or two in your deep state of relaxation to *appreciate* what you feel.

Day 15

With each breath, say to yourself *8 times each*

My arms and legs are heavy and warm.
My heartbeat is calm and regular.
My breathing is relaxed and comfortable.
My abdomen is warm.
My forehead is cool.
My mind is quiet and still.

Day 16—Pulse Localization

With each slow breath in, say to yourself

I feel the pulse in my face.

As you breathe out, *feel* mentally for the pulsation of your heartbeat and notice that the area becomes warmer. Repeat 4 times. Continue, saying 4 times each

I feel the pulse in my ...

Neck and throat	**Pelvis**
Chest	**Back**
Hands and fingers	**Legs**
Arms	**Feet and toes**
Abdomen	

Always terminate with a deep breath and a stretch.

Day 17

As you breathe in, say to yourself

I see and feel my feet expanding one inch in all directions.

As you breathe out, feel, "see," and experience a pleasant, light expansion like a "halo." Repeat 4 times for each area as you proceed.

I see and feel my_____expanding one inch in all directions.

Legs	**Shoulders**
Thighs	**Arms**
Abdomen	**Hands**
Lower back	**Neck**
Chest	**Head**

Pause for three or four breaths, then say and feel

I allow my entire body to return to normal size but remain deeply relaxed.

Day 18

As you breathe in, say to yourself

I see and feel my feet expanding *one* inch in all directions.

Repeat 4 times—as yesterday. Then

I see and feel my feet expanding *twelve* inches in all directions.

As you breathe out, feel, "see," and experience a 12-inch halo of light, pleasant expansion. Repeat 4 times for each area:

Legs	Shoulders
Thighs	Arms
Abdomen	Hands
Lower back	Neck
Chest	Head

Pause for three or four breaths, then say and feel

I allow my entire body to return to normal size but remain deeply relaxed.

Day 19

For 10 minutes focus your total attention on a watch or clock. Try to keep your mind focused *only* on the watch without allowing any other thought to wander in.

Day 20

Spend three minutes relaxing while coordinating with your breathing the phrase

I am relaxed.

Then project yourself to your own ideal place for relaxation. Choose a peaceful, totally natural site. Allow your mind to wander pleasantly in your idyllic spot for another seven minutes.

Day 21

Choose your favorite soft, dreamy music. Close your eyes. Breathe slowly and deeply and try to float with the music for 5 or 10 minutes.

Day 22

With each complete breath, say to yourself

Every day in every way I am getting better and better. [40 times]

Day 23

With each complete breath, say to yourself

Every day in every way I am becoming more and more healthy. [40 times]

Day 24

With each complete breath, say to yourself

I am free of all outside forces. [40 times]

Day 25

With each complete breath, say to yourself

I use my own consciousness to be free of all outside forces. [40 times]

Day 26

With each complete breath, say to yourself

I have everything within myself to enjoy every minute of every day. [40 times]

Day 27

With each complete breath, say to yourself

I am responsible for my thoughts and actions. [40 times]

Day 28

With each complete breath, say to yourself

I accept myself completely here and now. [40 times]

Day 29

With each complete breath, say to yourself

I am filled with loving kindness. [40 times]

Day 30

With each complete breath, say to yourself

I feel loving compassion for all other human beings. [40 times]

Day 31

With each complete breath, say to yourself

I am attuned to my highest spiritual goals. [40 times]

Day 32

With each complete breath, say to yourself

I am filled with universal love. [40 times]

Day 33

Review the first 32 days and use the technique that most appeals to you.

Day 34

Combine three of the techniques doing each about half as long as originally and extending the entire exercise at least 15 minutes.

Day 35

As you breathe, say to yourself

As I breathe in I collect all the tension in my feet.

As I breathe out I breathe out and let go all the tension in my feet.

Repeat twice for each area:

Legs	Abdomen	Entire Body
Thighs	Chest	
Hips	Arms	
Buttocks	Hands	
Pelvis	Neck and Throat	
Back	Head and Face	

You now have a variety of techniques for achieving and maintaining 10 to 15 minutes of deep relaxation. Practice at least one technique every day. Some days you may wish to try three separate techniques or combine different ones to help you. Select the one most effective for you. During Days 36 through 39 experiment on your own until you feel comfortable with a routine.

Now, while you continue your training sessions, let's pause to discuss some popular concepts of health and disease.

FIVE

Nutrition

GETTING DOWN TO THE LITTLE WE DO KNOW

Whether you have followed the daily programs for 40 days or are reading for the first time straight through, if you are concerned with health, you are probably already aware (you should be) of the importance of nutrition. Food is surely one of the favorite topics of conversation among Americans, though probably more confused than any other aspect of health. Relatively little scientific research has been done in the field, and the truly important cross-correlations suggested by some researchers have not yet been fully examined scientifically.

About all we do know for certain is that foods contain fats, carbohydrates, proteins, vitamins, and minerals, and that some sort of balance of all these elements is essential for good health.

For instance, in spite of the widespread publicity of the past twenty years, we are still uncertain of the best combination of fats. Although excess animal fats probably are harmful, there is now some evidence that man-made, artificially hydrogenated fats may be worse than animal fats. Margarine has been demonstrated to cause more hardening of the arteries than butter, at least in some research. So, first of all, I recommend that you *avoid artificially hydrogenated* or "partially hardened" fats. Try to maintain a ratio of 3 parts unsaturated fat to 2 parts saturated fat. In this respect pork lard is much better than most artificially hardened vegetable shortenings. Eggs, in spite of an ill-deserved reputation as having too much cholesterol, are also an excellent source of balanced fat: The ratio of polyunsaturated fats nicely exceeds that of saturated fats. The small quantity of cholesterol in eggs is insignificant compared with that manufactured by the body every day.

In carbohydrates the greatest bug is sugar, sucrose. Until 125 years ago, sugar was practically unused. Today it represents an average of 20 percent of calories consumed in this country, when sugar should make up no more than 5 percent, or preferably less, of one's total intake of calories. Other than this, the biggest problem with carbohydrates is our tendency to consume them in excess.

Protein is another essential to good health. About 70 to 100 grams of protein per day is recommended. But protein varies tremendously in its quality, that is its content of essential amino acids, of which human beings must have a good balance. Few vegetable proteins, for instance, except soybeans, are adequately balanced. However, those can be balanced by combining two or more complementary proteins, such as rice and beans. The best-quality protein comes from fish, eggs, milk and other dairy products, meat, soybeans, and nuts (except for peanuts), and seeds. *Diet for a Small Planet,* by Frances M. Lappé, is an excellent source of information about complementary proteins. Protein needs are greater in children than in adults, so it is especially important that children have a proper protein balance.

The idea of bran as a "preventive" for many diseases is gaining considerable support from such eminent physicians as Dr. Denis Burkett. Dr. Burkett felt that coronary artery disease, diverticulosis, appendicitis, gallstones, cancer and polyps of the colon and rectum, hemorrhoids, varicose veins, and obesity are all contributed to by the lack of adequate fiber in the American diet.*

A certain amount of bulk *is* essential, particularly for proper excretion of bile and good bowel motility. Diverticulosis may result more often from lack of bulk in the diet than any other cause. Whole grains, fruits, coarse vegetables, and so on provide bulk. But to ensure adequate fiber, ideally everyone should eat 3 to 9 tablespoons of bran daily. Experience will help you decide.

Very few diets that include a good balance of proteins, carbohydrates, and fats are deficient in minerals. Iodized or sea salt should be used *in moderation*. Total daily consumption of salt should not exceed 5 grams, as excessive intake of salt leads to greater and greater risk of high blood pressure and strokes. Hypertensive patients consume more than 4 times as much salt as do those with normal blood pressure.†

One of the very important sources of minerals is water. Today, however, many major cities have such heavily polluted water sources, reeking with chlorine, that we may soon have to resort to bottled spring water, as is essential in most of Europe. Although fluoride is useful in preventing dental decay and possibly in avoiding rarefaction of the bone, the quantity in some city water is probably larger than necessary. There is also the suspicion that bursitis may be aggravated by large intakes of fluorides. Of equally dangerous concern is artificially softened water, first because of its excess of salt, but, more importantly, because cadmium, a potentially harmful substance, has replaced zinc, a useful mineral. In short, don't drink artificially softened water. You may wish to choose a distiller. (Best ones in my opinion are available from Pure Water Society, P. O. Box 83226, Lincoln, Nebraska 68501.)

Although little significant work has been done on those ever present preservatives BHA and BHT, we

AMA News, Oct. 28, 1974, p. 16.
†Paul J. Schechter et al., "Sodium Chloride Preference in Essential Hypertension," *JAMA* 225 (1973): 1311–1315.

can say that they are such potent metabolic poisons that they can only be used in really minute quantities. Ideally we should avoid them, but it is probably more harmful to be worried constantly about the dangers of the chemicals than it is to consume them in limited quantities!

As far as vitamins are concerned, if you raised most of your own food, you probably wouldn't need to worry at all. But, if your food is overprocessed or has lain for days or weeks in a store, for example, you may need vitamin supplementation. Good daily supplies for adults are:

> *Vitamin A—10,000 to 25,000 units (avoid 50,000 units, which can be very harmful)*

> *Vitamin, B_1, B_2, and B_6—5 to 25 mg. of each*

> *Vitamin C—1 gram. There is a difference between natural C and "ascorbic acid"; it's the bioflavanoids—absent in ascorbic acid—that chemically and metabolically enhance Vitamin C's activity. Smoking more than a pack a day decreases the serum Vitamin C level by 40 percent.**

> *Vitamin E—400 units for women, 800 units for men. Men especially must avoid 1500 units or more, as so large an intake can be "feminizing."*

At a recent meeting, Dr. Daniel B. Menzel reported that Vitamin E in dosages 6 times that recommended by the F.D.A. helped protect against the stress of air pollutants.† If you live in polluted air, use 800 units daily.

Probably no other vitamin supplementation is likely to be needed except in special circumstances.

In summary, the following dietary recommendations can be made. Study them in combination with the accompanying charts of the carbohydrate content in different foods.

---

*Medical Tribune, Nov. 13, 1974.
†Vitamin Information Bureau Seminar in Chicago, reported in Hospital Tribune, Dec. 8, 1975.

Avoid completely, if possible:

1. *Processed foods (mixes, white flour, processed rice, dried potatoes, and so on).*

2. *Sugar.*

3. *Nicotine.*

4. *Caffeine (Coffee, tea, cocoa, colas).*

5. *Artificially hydrogenated fats (margarine, smooth peanut butter, cream substitutes).*

6. *Chlorinated water.*

7. *BHA, BHT, nitrates, and nitrites.*

Go light on:

1. *Any liquid with meals. Between meals drink juices, pure water, and herb teas.*

2. *Fats in meat, especially beef fat.*

3. *Milk (in adults).*

4. *Fruits (see the accompanying chart for fruits' carbohydrate content).*

Eat freely:

1. *Bran—1 to 3 ounces per day, as determined by regularity.*

2. *Meats—fish and poultry contain the most quality protein; then lamb, pork, and beef.*

3. *Eggs—one or two a day are good for you.*

4. *Butter—ideally mix 4 parts butter with 2 to 3 parts safflower or corn oil in a blender. Eat 4 ounces a day if desired.*

5. *Vegetables—see the carbohydrate list.*

6. *Pimma yogurt—get a culture and prepare your own. (Just set the culture mixed with whole milk at room temperature for 12 to 24 hours. Pimma*

CARBOHYDRATE CONTENT OF FRUITS AND VEGETABLES

Eat these preferably

3%	6%	9%	12%	15%	18%	21%
VEGETABLES:	VEGETABLES:	VEGETABLES:	VEGETABLES:	VEGETABLES:	VEGETABLES:	VEGETABLES:
Asparagus	Beans, green	Artichokes	Soybeans, dry	Beans, red	Horseradish	Beans, lima,
Beet greens	Beans, wax	Beets		Kidney beans,	Potatoes	fresh
Broccoli	Eggplant	Brussels	FRUITS:	canned		Corn, fresh
Cabbage	Leeks	sprouts	Apricots	Parsnips	FRUITS:	
Cauliflower	Okra	Carrots	Cherries, sour	Peas	Cherries,	FRUITS:
Celery	Parsley	Onions	Loganberries		sweet	Bananas
Cucumber	Pepper, green	Rutabagas	Oranges	FRUITS:	Crabapples	Prunes
Lettuce	Pepper, red		Peaches	Apples	Figs, fresh	
Mustard	Pumpkin	FRUITS:	Pineapple	Blueberries	Pomegranates	
greens	Squash,	Blackberries	Plums	Grapes		
Radishes	winter	Cranberries	Raspberries	Huckleberries		
Sauerkraut	Turnips	Currants		Mangos		
Spinach		Gooseberries		Nectarines		
Squash,	FRUITS:	Grapefruit		Pears		
summer	Cantaloupe	Lemons				
Tomatoes	Honeydew	Limes				
Turnip tops	Strawberries	Tangerines				
	Watermelon					

mixed thoroughly with fresh fruits is an ideal dessert.)

7. Nuts and seeds—the most nourishing are almonds, pecans, walnuts, sunflower seeds, pumpkin and squash seeds. (Dry them in the oven with a little butter and very little salt.)

If you are not raising your own fresh vegetables, especially salads, then by all means supplement with vitamins as listed earlier in the chapter.

If even after you correct your diet you still don't feel healthy, ask your physician to do a hair analysis for possible trace mineral imbalances, by sending a hair sample to Analytico Laboratories, 100 East Cheyenne Road, Colorado Springs, Colorado; or Bio-Medical Data, Inc., Box 66907, Chicago, A.M.F., O'Hare, Illinois 60666.

Deficiencies of zinc, chromium, magnesium, and manganese are very common. If you need supplements of those, be sure they are chemically bonded to soybean proteins to make them more usable in the body. They may be ordered from The Chemins Company, 2430 Mesa Road, Colorado Springs, Colorado 80904, or Lanpar Company, Box 35227, Dallas, Texas 75235.

In general, however, mineral analyses and supplements should be ordered only under the supervision of a physician. For instance, did you know that alcohol and meat both increase the need for magnesium, but sugar acts to inhibit its absorption? Or that calcium competes with magnesium for absorption? As you can see, achieving correct mineral balance is tremendously complicated, and requires the knowledge and experience of a doctor preferably a specialist in nutrition. But always keep in mind, too, that *emotional tension and stress are probably more harmful than any food.*

If you think you don't eat much sugar, look at this! The following list shows the approximate amounts of refined sugar (that is added sugar in addition to the sugar naturally present) "hidden" in popular foods.

Food Item	Size Portion	Approximate Sugar Content In Teaspoonfuls Of Granulated Sugar
BEVERAGES		
cola drinks	1 (6 oz bottle or glass)	3½
cordials	1 (¾ oz glass)	1½
ginger ale	6 oz	5
highball	1 (6 oz glass)	2½
orangeade	1 (8 oz glass)	5
root beer	1 (10 oz bottle)	4½
Seven-Up®	1 (6 oz bottle or glass)	3¾
soda pop	1 (8 oz bottle)	5
sweet cider	1 cup	6
whiskey sour	1 (3 oz glass)	1½
CAKES AND COOKIES		
angel food	1 (4 oz piece)	7
apple sauce cake	1 (4 oz piece)	5½
banana cake	1 (2 oz piece)	2
cheese cake	1 (4 oz piece)	2
choc. cake (plain)	1 (4 oz piece)	6
choc. cake (iced)	1 (4 oz piece)	10
coffee cake	1 (4 oz piece)	4½
cup cake (iced)	1	6
fruit cake	1 (4 oz piece)	5
jelly roll	1 (2 oz piece)	2½
orange cake	1 (4 oz piece)	4
pound cake	1 (4 oz piece)	5
sponge cake	1 (1 oz piece)	2
brownies (unfrosted)	1 (¾ oz)	3
chocolate cookies	1	1½
Fig Newtons®	1	5
gingersnaps	1	3
macaroons	1	6
nut cookies	1	1½
oatmeal cookies	1	2
sugar cookies	1	1½
chocolate eclair	1	7
cream puff	1	2
donut (plain)	1	3
donut (glazed)	1	6

Food Item	Size Portion	Approximate Sugar Content In Teaspoonfuls Of Granulated Sugar
CANDIES		
average choc. milk bar	1 (1½ oz)	2½
chewing gum	1 stick	½
chocolate cream	1 piece	2
butterscotch chew	1 piece	1
chocolate mints	1 piece	2
fudge	1 oz square	4½
gumdrop	1	2
hard candy	4 oz	20
Lifesavers®	1	⅓
peanut brittle	1 oz	3½
CANNED FRUITS AND JUICES		
canned apricots	4 halves and 1 T syrup	3½
canned fruit juices (sweet)	½ cup	2
canned peaches	2 halves and 1 T syrup	3½
fruit salad	½ cup	3½
fruit syrup	2 T	2½
stewed fruits	½ cup	2
DAIRY PRODUCTS		
ice cream	⅓ pt (3½ oz)	3½
ice cream cone	1	3½
ice cream soda	1	5
ice cream sundae	1	7
malted milk shake	1 (10 oz glass)	5
JAMS AND JELLIES		
apple butter	1 T	1
jelly	1 T	4–6
orange marmalade	1 T	4–6
peach butter	1 T	1
strawberry jam	1 T	4

Food Item	Size Portion	Approximate Sugar Content In Teaspoonfuls Of Granulated Sugar
DESSERTS, MISCELLANEOUS		
apple cobbler	½ cup	3
blueberry cobbler	½ cup	3
custard	½ cup	2
fresh pastry	1 (4 oz piece)	5
fruit gelatin	½ cup	4½
apple pie	1 slice (average)	7
apricot pie	1 slice	7
berry pie	1 slice	10
butterscotch pie	1 slice	4
cherry pie	1 slice	10
cream pie	1 slice	4
lemon pie	1 slice	7
mince meat pie	1 slice	4
peach pie	1 slice	7
prune pie	1 slice	6
pumpkin pie	1 slice	5
rhubarb pie	1 slice	4
banana pudding	½ cup	2
bread pudding	½ cup	1½
chocolate pudding	½ cup	4
cornstarch pudding	½ cup	2½
date pudding	½ cup	7
fig pudding	½ cup	7
Grapenut® pudding	½ cup	2
plum pudding	½ cup	4
rice pudding	½ cup	5
tapioca pudding	½ cup	3
berry tart	1 cup	10
blancmange	½ cup	5
brown Betty	½ cup	3
plain pastry	1 (4 oz piece)	3
sherbet	½ cup	9
SYRUPS, SUGARS, AND ICINGS		
brown sugar	1 T	*3
chocolate icing	1 oz	5
chocolate sauce	1 T	3½

Food Item	Size Portion	Approximate Sugar Content In Teaspoonfuls Of Granulated Sugar
SYRUPS, SUGARS, AND ICINGS (continued)		
corn syrup	1 T	*3
granulated sugar	1 T	*3
honey	1 T	*3
Karo® syrup	1 T	*3
maple syrup	1 T	*5
molasses	1 T	*3½
white icing	1 oz	*5

*Actual sugar content

This chapter's purpose has been to inspire you to revise your diet to include healthy foods and to omit the bad ones, or, if you are overweight, to convince you to make a real effort to lose weight slowly (¼ to ⅓ pound per day) down to your ideal weight. Likewise, if you smoke, or drink excessively, it is hoped that you will work specifically to overcome your unhealthy habits. In fact, whatever your undesirable or unhealthy habits, now is the time to give them up. So, if appropriate, during the next week use one or more of the habit-regulating techniques of the next chapter.

SIX

Habit Regulation

Almost any habit can be controlled if one has a desire to do so and is willing to practice the exercises necessary for the mental retraining. Four examples of habit regulation are (1) weight control, (2) freedom from smoking, (3) freedom from alcohol, and (4) learning to sleep better. Other habits may be substituted in similar mental exercise programs.

Days 40 Through 47

During Days 40 through 47, concentrate on the appropriate exercise from among the following. Read the exercise 6 times and practice at least 3 times a day.

WEIGHT BALANCE

Read 6 times, then practice.
Spend 5 minutes entering a state of deep relaxation (use your favorite technique).

Now I see myself and feel myself as perfectly healthy and happy. And I project myself to my own private, perfect room, my own hideaway where I can happily go to know myself. I see myself enter and close the door. My room is furnished

ideally for my desires. I undress and look at my body in my own full-length mirror. [*Pause one minute.*] I see my body just as realistically as anything I've ever seen.

Now I visualize and feel my body at my ideal weight. [*Pause 2 minutes.*]

My appetite is pleasantly satisfied. [*10 times*]

I visualize and feel my body at my ideal weight.

I become increasingly comfortable as I attain my desired weight [*3 times*]

I become healthier and healthier as I attain my desired weight [*3 times*]

I feel increasing pride and joy as I attain my desired weight.

I am attuned with my highest self, lovingly and happily.

My appetite is pleasantly satisfied. I am satisfied with just enough calories to maintain my ideal weight. [*10 times*]

I visualize and feel my body at my ideal weight. And I will carry this image and feeling with me as I return to normal awareness.

Now as I prepare to return to my normal awareness, I feel myself bringing with me the health, happiness, and love I feel and see. I take a deep breath, open my eyes, and stretch comfortably, feeling satisfied and filled with loving energy.

If you have difficulty remembering all the phrases, pick out the one or two most meaningful to you and repeat them 10 to 20 times. At the same time, create a vision of yourself standing on a scale which shows you at your ideal weight.

If you're overweight practice this technique three times *every day,* preferably before each meal. If you're underweight, you can benefit in the same way.

FREEDOM FROM SMOKING

Read 6 times, then choose one or two of the phrases and say each 10 to 20 times.

Spend 5 minutes entering your deepest state of relaxation, then repeat—

Now I visualize myself as satisfied and free from smoking.

Each day I become less dependent on smoking.

I become healthier and healthier as I smoke less.

I become more and more comfortable as I smoke less.

I visualize myself as satisfied and free from smoking.

I feel increasing pride and joy as I accomplish my goal.

I am calm and relaxed and free from smoking.

Now as I prepare to return to my normal awareness, I feel myself bringing with me the health, happiness, and love I feel and see. I take a deep breath, pleasantly open my eyes, stretch my body comfortably and feel myself filled with loving energy.

Continue practicing every day until you are comfortably weaned from smoking. Any time you feel the need to smoke repeat this exercise.

FREEDOM FROM ALCOHOL

Read 6 times; choose one or two phrases and repeat each 10 to 20 times after you have spent 5 minutes reaching a deep level of relaxation.

Now I visualize myself as satisfied and free of alcohol.

Each day I abstain for longer and longer periods of time.

I become more and more comfortable as I become free of alcohol.

I gain increasing benefits as I become free of alcohol.

I am attuned with my highest self, lovingly and happily.

I visualize myself as satisfied and free of alcohol.

I feel increasing pride as I accomplish my goal.

I am calm and relaxed and free of alcohol.

Now as I prepare to return to my normal awareness, I feel myself bringing with me the health, happiness, and love I feel and see. I take a deep breath, pleasantly open my eyes, and stretch all the muscles of my body, feeling myself filled with loving energy.

Practice at least three times daily and wean yourself from alcohol over two to four weeks. Substitute this mental exercise anytime you feel the need for a drink.

SLEEP HARMONY

Read 6 times, then enter a deep state of relaxation. Continue repeating one or more of the following phrases until you fall asleep.

Now I visualize myself resting perfectly comfortably. I am relaxing deeper and deeper. I am proceeding deeper and deeper toward normal, restful sleep. [*Pause 30 seconds. Repeat 4 times and then wait one minute.*]   ..

I imagine myself lying in my perfect place of relaxation.

I am more and more deeply relaxed. [*Repeat 4 times.*]

I am at peace. [*Repeat 4 times.*]

I will now fall pleasantly asleep and awaken re-freshed at whatever hour I choose [*Specify the hour.*] And I keep repeating "I am deeper and deeper relaxed" until I fall asleep.

For practice, one might specify 10 to 15 minutes, then, after a period of relaxation at this deeper level of awareness—

I will return to my normal level of conscious-ness, bringing with me the rest and relaxation that I have experienced. As I take another deep, pleasant breath, I open my eyes and look around, stretching my entire body, and feeling myself com-pletely refreshed and filled with energy.

If you program yourself every night for a month, you should never again have difficulty falling asleep.

After Days 40 through 47, continue to practice your habit-regulation technique at least once or twice daily. Now, while you concentrate on overcoming your undesirable habits, let's continue our overview of health with a look at physical exercise.

SEVEN

Physical Exercise

Most of us, whether we pay attention to it or not, realize that physical exercise is essential for health. But we must remember that two criteria must be met if the full benefits of exercise are to be realized: (1) Limbering must be sufficient to keep all joints, muscles, and tendons at normal flexibility; and (2) The exercise must be strenuous enough to provide strengthening of the heart.

Limbering can be maintained through a daily 10-to-15-minute exercise similar to that developed for our patients at the Pain Rehabilitation Center. These exercises are simple, safe, and reasonable for almost everyone.

If you are forty or over, or if you are thirty-five or over and smoke, you should have a stress EKG done before beginning the Aerobics—the cardiac strengthening exercises.

The number of times the following exercise is tolerated will be determined by your physical ability. Begin with a minimum of two or three repetitions of each exercise and add one each day. When you become tired or short of breath, rest, and then proceed. The exercises may be adapted to individual needs whenever necessary. Do a complete set of exercises in consecutive order at least twice a day. At least one of those times, try one of the relaxation techniques *after* physical exercise, just to experience the tremendous revitalization you will achieve from both practices. Hopefully, you will begin these exercises early in your health program and stay with them for life.

1. Head Rolls

Starting Position: Stand or sit erect. Allow arms to hang loose at your sides.

Action: Gently drop chin to chest and roll head to the right in a full circle. Repeat this to the left. Work up to 10 in each direction.

Purpose: To relieve a stiff or aching neck or a headache and to remain limber.

2. Shoulders Up and Down

Starting Position: Stand or sit erect. Allow arms to hang loosely at your sides (Position 1).

Action: Bring shoulders up toward your ears as far as possible (Position 2), then as far back as possible, pulling the shoulder blades together in the back. Relax to starting position. Do this in a circular motion. Keep head erect and neck straight. Work up to 20 times.

Purpose: To loosen up the muscles of the shoulders and neck.

3. Wing Stretcher

Starting Position: Stand erect, elbows at shoulder height, fists clenched in front of chest, or fingertips touching.

Action: Thrust elbows vigorously backward without arching back. Keep head erect, elbows at shoulder height. Return to starting position. Work up to 20 times.

Purpose: To stretch the chest muscles to improve posture.

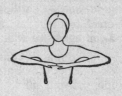

4. Arm Circles

Starting Position: Stand erect, arms extended sideways at shoulder height, palms up.

Action: Describe large circles backward with hands. Reverse. Turn palms down, do small circles forward. Work up to 20 of each.

Purpose: To loosen up the muscles of the shoulders, shoulder blades, and upper back.

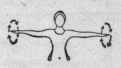

5. Sitting Stretch

Starting Position: Sit on floor or mat, spread legs apart, place hands on knees (Position 1).

Action: Bend forward at waist, extending arms as far down legs as possible, reaching for toes (Position 2). Return to starting position and repeat. Work up to 20 times.

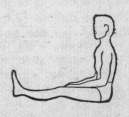

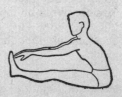

Purpose: To stretch the muscles of the inner thigh and back of the knee.

6. Knee-ups

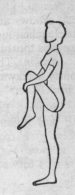

Starting Position: Stand erect, feet together, arms at sides. Lean against a wall if necessary.

Action: Raise left knee as high as possible, grasping leg below knee and pulling knee against body. Keep back straight. Lower to starting position. Repeat with right leg. Work up to 10 of each.

Purpose: Provides excellent exercise for sacroiliac joint.

7. Sitting Knee Stretch

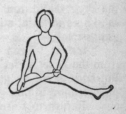

Starting Position: Sit erect on floor or mat. Legs should be straight and shoulder-width apart.

Action: Bring right foot to top of left thigh with left hand. Press right knee to floor with right hand as far as possible. Release pressure and repeat. Reverse to left leg. Work up to 10 with each leg.

Purpose: Another excellent sacroiliac and hip-joint exercise; helps mobility of these joints.

8. Body Bender

Starting Position: Stand, feet shoulder-width apart, hands behind neck, fingers interlaced.

Action: Bend trunk sideways to the right as far as possible, keeping hands behind neck. Return to starting position. Repeat to the left. Do not bend forward or backward, only to the side. Work up to 10 in each direction.

Purpose: To stretch and strengthen the muscles and joints along the sides of the spine.

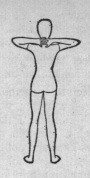

9. Hip Walks

Starting Position: Sit on floor, legs slightly separated and out straight in front of you.

Action: Walk on your seat 10 moves forward and 10 backward.

Purpose: To exercise the waist and hips.

10. Slow Down

Starting Position: Kneel on the floor. Hold your body from the knees up in as straight a line as possible.

Action: Lean backward from the knees as far as you can. Put both hands on your heels or on the floor behind you for balance. Return to starting position and repeat. Work up to 20.

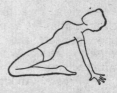

Purpose: Stretches and strengthens the thigh muscles and the arch of the lumbar spine. It should not be attempted by those with significant back problems.

11. Jogging in Place

Action: Run or hop in place, raising feet as high off the floor as possible. Slowly taper off speed so body function returns to normal.

12. Side Body Bender

Starting Position: Stand with feet slightly farther apart than shoulder width, arms loose at sides.

Action: Step to side with right foot and point it directly outward to the right. Bend right knee. Bend body to the right, sliding right arm as far down the right leg as possible. Return to the starting position and repeat. This may be done in a bouncing action, in which case you do not return to the starting position until you are ready to repeat to the left. Work up to 10 times with each leg.

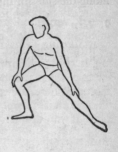

Purpose: Stretches and strengthens thighs and hips.

13. The Bridge

Starting Position: Lie on your back with your knees bent and feet flat on the floor.

Action: Lift buttocks straight into the air and *hold*—for 15 seconds at first, working up gradually to 5 minutes.

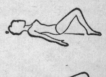

Purpose: Strengthens back muscles. If you also lift your head off the floor leaving only shoulders, upper back, and feet on the floor, additional benefit is gained.

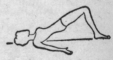

CARDIOVASCULAR STRENGTHENING

Exercise that adequately strengthens the heart must increase pulse rate. People unaccustomed to exercise and those over forty should begin these programs cautiously and slowly. The programs outlined in *New Aerobics* by Colonel Kenneth Cooper and *Aerobics for Women* by Colonel Cooper and his wife are so superior to anything else I've seen that I recommend them very highly. Be sure you start with the tests suggested, choose a specific progressive program, and follow it to increasing energy and health.

Supervised physical exercise has been known to help lower blood pressure both in normal people and in those with high blood pressure. Any way you look at it, physical exercise, both limbering and strengthening, is vital to health. Every day of your life you should include some planned exercise such as the programs discussed here, unless you are one of the few Americans who exercises *adequately and regularly,* at work or play. If you are, continue!

EIGHT

Emotions and Health

Emotions and moods vary tremendously. They are affected by heredity and especially by the home environment. But chemical influences, especially diet, light, physical exercise, and habits, all strongly influence emotions. While you're still working on those habits, consider the following self-tests. Ask yourself these questions:

Do I get irritable, annoyed, angry, or depressed when—

1. *I don't have adequate sleep.*

2. *I feel as if I'm being attacked unfairly.*

3. *I'm under any stress.*

4. *I'm surrounded by people.*

5. *I'm out of the limelight.*

6. *I lose, even in a simple game.*

7. *I'm around other disturbed persons.*

8. *I have to compromise on my desires.*

9. *I'm held up by someone being late.*

10. *I'm by myself.*

11. *I have to watch my temper.*

12. *I have to get up in the morning.*

13. *I'm not perfectly dressed.*

14. *I can't have that quick drink in the evening (or earlier).*

15. *The weather is bad.*

16. *There's a lot of noise.*

17. *I can't smoke.*

18. *Someone else smokes near me.*

19. *I drive.*

20. *I have any crisis in life.*

21. *I have to meet new people.*

22. *I'm criticized.*

23. *I have to go to a social function.*

24. *I have to go to a doctor or dentist.*

25. *I make an error.*

If you answer yes to more than 8 of the questions, you need to balance your own emotions more effectively; if you answer yes to more than 15 of them, you're in real trouble emotionally. Slow down. Take a look at where you've been and where you're going. Spend a few minutes thinking about and writing your answers to these questions:

What are your goals?

What is worthwhile in life?

What problems deserve your attention or concern?

According to Dr. Meyer Friedman and Dr. R. H. Rosenman, authors of *Type A Behavior and Your*

Heart, people who are compulsive "workaholics"—Type A personality, they label it—are very prone to develop coronary artery disease or to have heart attacks. Indeed, emotional distress is far more implicated in heart disease than diet, exercise, or any other aspect of life so far intelligently and scientifically studied.

Type A people have an intense sense of urgency. They do everything with great haste but never find enough time to do all the things that are planned. Similarly, they are always impatient with the snail's pace at which everyone *else* is working. Others talk too slowly, work too slowly, and even play too slowly for Type A's. For them, waiting in line is particularly stressful. The Type A is truely the "Speedy Gonzalez" of the business world.

Most likely, the Type A personality has a great deal of hostility. His competition is of an angry nature. He always seems to be riled in arguments, games, and business. He probably has an explosive speech pattern, or a habit such as clenching his fists or jaws, or grinding his teeth.

Type A people have difficulty restricting mental activity to a single thought. They read while eating, and while thinking about one problem they are likely to be distracted by a dozen others at the same time.

Type A's, who incidentally tend to be men more often than women, are particularly upset and feel guilty when they have nothing to do.

Despite all this intensity and speed, the Type A person never has any time to do those things that are really fun and really count in life. The following is a test you may use to determine which of the two personality types you are. Obviously, there are other criteria, also.

How do you decide if you're a Type A or Type B person? Try these for size:

1. *I'm always busy, even if it's just wiggling or doodling.*

2. *I smoke.*

3. *I often feel ill when I have a deadline.*

4. *I chew my fingernails.*

5. *New people make me nervous.*

6. *I hate pokey drivers.*

7. *I get very irritable if I have to wait.*

8. *I'm always in a hurry.*

9. *I can hear my heart beating and it often skips a beat.*

10. *I gulp my meals.*

11. *I have trouble going to sleep.*

12. *I have to chew gum or something else.*

13. *I have to take a drink or a sleeping pill at night.*

14. *I lose my temper easily.*

15. *I need a drink to relax.*

16. *I am apt to be nauseated, dizzy, or faint or have cramps when I'm stressed.*

17. *I fiddle with my hair, scratch a lot, or pick my nose.*

18. *I get upset easily.*

19. *I don't like to watch other people talk.*

20. *Noises irritate me a lot.*

21. *I prefer active sports.*

22. *I have to talk a lot when I'm around other people.*

23. *I worry a lot.*

24. *I'm impatient with others.*

25. *I can't sit still; I have to have something to do.*

If you have over 14 "yes" answers you lean toward Type A, and if you have 20 to 25 yes answers, start right away to learn to slow down. Remember, the type B personality lives longer. It is important to recognize that the main problem with Type A personality is that it tends to wear out your heart by reacting so vigorously to the stress of life. Many "A" characteristics, in moderation, seem socially desirable. Type B persons might be considered lazy by the "A's," but a well-motivated "B" will often outdistance the more intensely competitive Type A. Through Biogenics we can all work to become relaxed, happy, productive human beings.

Here are some more questions for testing your ability to endure stress:

1. Are you upset—

by stress?

by inadequate sleep?

by having too many people around?

by having no one around?

if someone picks on you?

if you lose?

if you are ignored?

if you don't have an audience of admirers?

if you're held up and can't make a meeting?

if the weather is bad?

If you answer yes to seven or more of these, you're likely to be very uptight and really need to learn to relax and let go. Just think, is any one of those events really worth so much of your concern?

2. Are you—

confident of finances?

certain you had a good breakfast today?

likely to like most people?

feeling good physically?

feeling relaxed and happy?

getting adequate sleep?

feeling well adjusted?

If you can truthfully answer yes to five or more of these, you're likely to be in a secure emotional state— at least right now.

3. Do you really—

enjoy yourself?

like your body?

feel well coordinated?

feel attractive?

If your answer is yes to all these, you have a good self-image. If not, this book was written especially for you!

The regular practice of progressive physical exercise, both limbering and cardiovascular strengthening, and Biogenics exercises, is an ideal way to avoid "being recycled" earlier than is necessary.

Some additional recommendations are:

1. Chew slowly; *enjoy your meals. Take* at least *20 minutes to eat.*

2. Take time to relax 10 to 15 minutes three times each day.

3. Listen to soft, pleasant music.

4. Develop a habit of saying, "I am relaxed and comfortable," to yourself several times each hour.

5. Learn to recognize inner feelings of stress, and when you note them, close your eyes, take a deep breath several times, saying, "I am relaxed."

6. *Get plenty of physical exercise. Follow the Aerobics program.*

7. *Avoid working more than 10 hours a day.*

8. *Take off at least one and a half days each week (say, Saturday noon through Sunday) just for relaxation and fun. That old saying, "All work and no play . . . ," really is true. Too many Type A people work even on weekends. Develop the play habit.*

NINE

Advanced Biogenics®

Having learned how to relax, exercise physically, eat properly, and recognize your emotional strengths and weaknesses, you are now ready to begin a more in-depth training program designed to broaden your experience and pleasure. You may either do each of these exercises three times on the day indicated, or do it once and practice one of your earlier favorites, or habit regulation, the other two times.

Day 48

Relax. Take a deep, pleasant breath, then say and do the following with eyes open:

> I look around a bit and turn my head slightly to see my surroundings. I look and see but I don't judge. I don't comment on it; I just look. I look around. I see what is here. Now, as I look I observe only color. I ignore form. I concentrate on an individual color that I like. [*Focus 5 minutes.*]

> Now I concentrate on depth. I ignore color. I focus on depth, width, height. [*Focus 5 minutes.*]

Terminate in the usual way.

Day 49

Read twice, then do.

Relax, close your eyes, and experience the following—

I touch a piece of cloth with my fingers [*About one minute.*]

Now I stop touching but continue to *feel* the cloth with my mind. [*One to two minutes*.]

Do the same with your

Face

Arms

Chest

Abdomen

Legs

Then feel inside your mouth with your tongue, follow it by feeling with your mind. Complete by feeling your body as a whole before terminating.

Day 50

Relax, focus on breathing and relaxation for 3 minutes, then pick only one *pleasant* body sensation. Say the word for it over and over to yourself and spend 5 to 10 minutes concentrating only on that one sensation or feeling.

Day 51

Spend 3 minutes entering a deep state of relaxation. Then concentrate on a part of your body you dislike for some reason. Spend 10 to 12 minutes focusing on a feeling and vision of pure love filling and surrounding that part of your body.

Day 52

Relax. Then as you breathe in, say to yourself

I am aware of sensations coming to me from my environment.

As you breathe out, say to yourself

I am aware of myself as being part of those sensations.

Repeat 40 times.

Day 53

Obtain a bright red cloth or piece of paper.
Spend 5 minutes focusing on the color. Then close your eyes and try to see, feel, hear, taste, smell only red. Fill your consciousness with red.

Day 54

Repeat with orange.

Day 55

Repeat with yellow.

Day 56

Repeat with green (a bright forest or emerald green).

Day 57

Repeat with blue (be specific—choose royal blue, or navy).

Day 58

Repeat with violet.

Day 59

Repeat with white.

Day 60

Repeat with pink.

Day 61

Repeat using a live rosebud.

Day 62

With every breath, repeat to yourself

I am building a beautifully functioning body and mind. [40 times]

Day 63

With every breath, repeat to yourself

I know that my innermost being is magnificent—wise and loving. [40 times]

Day 64

With every breath, repeat to yourself

I love and appreciate the universal life force which sustains me. [40 times]

Day 65

With every breath, repeat to yourself

I am attuned to my highest spiritual goals. [40 times]

Day 66

Read, then do.

Sit and recall the three worst events of your life. Write them down. Then reexperience them as you say *aloud,* eyes closed

Pain—pain—pain—

Chant it, feel it. Repeat it for 3 to 5 minutes.

After 5 minutes, recall the pleasantest event of your life, and reexperience it as you say *aloud,* eyes closed

Love—love—love—

Continue for 3 to 5 minutes.

Day 67

Recall yesterday's three most unpleasant events. Now ask yourself

1. How much of those old negative problems do I still carry with me? [*Think about it one minute.*]

2. How much energy do I waste focusing on past negativity? [*Think about it one minute.*]

3. How much anger, fear, guilt, depression do I keep with me each day? [*Think about it one minute.*]

4. Am I ready to give it up? [*Think about it one minute.*]

Then repeat to yourself with each breath as you relax

I release into the hands of God all anger, fear, and depression. [20 times]

Day 68

As you breathe, repeat to yourself

I release into the hands of God all anger, fear, and depression.

I see and feel myself filled and surrounded by light and love. [20 times each]

Day 69

As you breathe, repeat to yourself

I see and feel myself filled and surrounded by light and love. [40 times]

Day 70

As you breathe, repeat to yourself

I forgive myself for all my past transgressions. [40 times]

Day 71

As you breathe, repeat to yourself

I forgive all other human beings for their errors and transgressions. [40 times]

Day 72

As you breathe in, repeat to yourself

Every thought is a prayer.

As you breathe out, repeat to yourself

**I pray only for love and peace.
[Repeat 40 times.]**

Day 73

Choose the most meaningful experience, good or bad, of the past ten years. Relax, then focus your attention vividly upon reliving the experience. If it was unpleasant, integrate it into your life by forgiving yourself and others. If it was pleasant, just enjoy again the pleasure of that experience.

Day 74

Repeat the exercise for the previous ten-year period.

Day 75

Repeat for the ten-year period before that.

Day 76

Repeat for any other memory of your life you wish to reexamine.

Day 77

Spend 30 seconds *squirming*—kicking, hitting, twisting—in all directions. Then relax 30 seconds. Repeat 10 times, winding up with 3 minutes of deep relaxation.

Day 78

Count down from your current age to zero, one count per complete deep, slow breath. When you reach zero, allow your mind to drift comfortably wherever it wishes for 3 minutes.

Day 79

Read, then do.

Spend 3 minutes relaxing. Project yourself to your ideal private room. Mentally undress and examine yourself in your mirror. Then imagine that you are changing to the opposite sex. Mentally examine your body, mind, emotions, and life style for 5 minutes. Then see yourself change back to your own sex and appreciate yourself for what you are.

Days 80, 81, and 82

Repeat as above, but see yourself change each day to a different skin color—white, black, yellow, reddish bronze. Try to reach emotionally to appreciate the personality of given races.

Day 83

Repeat as on Day 79, but see yourself change to the personality of your mother.

Day 84

Do the same for your father.

Day 85

Do the same for someone you dislike or with whom you have a problem. Before you end the session, forgive "yourself" in your new role for any past transgressions.

Day 86

Do the same for someone you love and admire.

Day 87

Read, then do.

Relax 3 minutes, then project yourself into the past. See yourself entering the most famous healing temple known to man.

Meet the priests and physicians. See yourself being perfectly healed.

Day 88

Read, then do.

Relax 3 minutes, then project yourself to a beautiful mountain. Climb the mountain, seeing and hearing all the events about you. At the top of the mountain, you will see a wise man. Go up, introduce yourself, become acquainted, and ask the wise man your most important questions. Listen carefully to his answers.

This exercise, called the "Wise Man Attunement" is expanded and elaborated in the chapter, "Guided Exercises."

Day 89

Read the excerpt from "Relaxation and Meditation" by Thomas Elbert Clemmons (who is one of my patients) at the end of this chapter. *Try to feel and see the images as you read.*

Day 90—First Session

Compose your own exercise, making sure to include in it the following points:

Relaxation

Balancing of body

Balancing of mind and emotions

Spiritual attunement

Do your exercise. Try it at least once with good inspirational music.

Day 90—Second Session

Read, then do.

Relax deeply for 5 minutes. Then project yourself to your ideal spot of relaxation. Shortly, as you rest there, you will see an unknown living being—man, woman, child, or animal. Allow the person or creature to approach, and introduce yourself. Learn the sex and name of your new acquaintance.

Discuss any problems with your new acquaintance. Ask for advice on your troubles, and answers to your questions. If you get no answer, send for another who can. Ask for, expect to receive, and receive help in solving your problem before terminating.

After Day 90

At some convenient time try the guided exercises later in this book. But *every* day do your normal practicing at least 3 times. Twice each day you may just do deep relaxation, coupled, if you like, with habit regulation or your specific health goal. Once each day, spend 20 or 30 minutes doing your own special creation as on Day 90. Notice the great variety of illuminating experiences you'll have.

RELAXATION AND MEDITATION
by *Thomas Elbert Clemmons*

. . . Later as this lad grew into manhood and into old age, he watched scienfists split the unsplittable atom and astronauts walk and talk on the moon, and he came to conceive of the God of the poet of the Judean hills and the Great Spirit of the Cherokee brave as being one and the same but not limited to the Carolina mountains or the Judean hills or even to the planet Earth, but permeating all the universes and all the galaxies. As he developed a fuller appreciation of the vastness of time and space, he became increasingly aware of the limitations of his own body and mind. With his arms he could reach a few feet. With his feet he could walk a few miles. With his eyes and ears he could see and hear clearly for a short distance. If he turned to his mind, his memory could take him back a few decades. With the help of historians, he could turn back the leaves of time a few centuries. The archaeologists and the anthropologists would take him back over a dim trail for a few millenniums, back into the misty past. But to the question, "And before that?" he heard only the echo of his own voice. He turned to the men with the microscopes, and they assured him that his body was composed of billions of living cells, perfectly formed and marvelously designed and so tiny that he could hold a billion in one hand. But he remembered that during his college days the atom was considered indivisible. Now it is composed of electrons, protons and neutrons and comparatively large spaces between, and he asked, "And the design of the cell?" but the microscope would not reveal the answer.

He turned to the men with the telescope realizing that with his naked eye he could see approximately two thousand stars, with Galileo and his crude telescope, several thousands. But Von Braun and Teller looking into a mighty telescope on Mt. Palomar assured him there were billions of stars in the galaxies, enough that every human being, man, woman and child, on the earth could own one had he only the means to possess it. He traveled with the astronauts through the universe, past the Milky Way and on to the Andromeda nebula. But when he asked, "And beyond the Andromeda nebula?" the mighty telescopes showed only the darkness and the void.

Feeling like the mariner who prayed:

Lord, I need Your help because my boat is so small and Your ocean so large,

he turned slowly from the men of science, the high priests of learning of our era.

Next, I turn to the philosophers where one of my favorite authors, the great Roman emperor and stoic philosopher, Marcus Aurelius, reminds me that I am not the author of my being, that the Master Playwright wrote the script, and determined whether it would be

one act or two acts or three acts and whether I would
be on stage for a moment or a longer period of time.
When I pause and realize that the Divine Playwright
has seen fit to let me strut across the stage of life for a
full life's span of three score years and ten I find it
easy to join with the Psalmist when he sings:

> Enter into His gates with thanksgiving
> and into His courts with praise.

To have been permitted to play through the entire
three acts in the mighty drama of humanity and the
galaxies during the most exciting period in history
makes me very humble and grateful and ready to appreciate Marcus Aurelius' advice when he said:

> The Author of your being determined when you
> would enter the stage, and He will give you the
> cue for your departure; therefore, depart cheer-
> fully.

Knowing that in a few years I will receive this signal, I
glance toward the exit, where I see a number of doors.
The inscription over the first was written by the great
Persian poet, Omar Khayyam. It reads:

> The flower that once has bloomed forever dies.

I look back on the long hard depression days when I
traveled the Tennessee hills. After a long and strenuous
day filled with exertion and excitement a way-side inn
and a night of restful sleep were most inviting. So if
the Great Playwright has planned this exit for me, a
deep and dreamless sleep without pain, without problems, without worry or concern would be as welcome
as a featherbed on a cold winter night.

As I contemplate this eternity of ease a second
door appears surrounded by Grecian columns. Here
the quotation which is taken from Socrates, whom
Plato called the wisest of men, reads:

> *I am quite ready to acknowledge that I ought to be grieved at death if I were not persuaded that I am going to other gods who are wise and good (of this I am as certain as I can be of any such matters) and to men departed who are better than those whom I leave behind.*

If Socrates is correct this would indeed be an exciting adventure—to meet the great men who have gone before, to listen to Socrates as he talked of *the good and the true and the beautiful,* to travel the middle way with the great Buddha in search of *enlightenment,* to learn much of *conduct and character* and respect for age and authority from Confucius, to walk by the Sea of Galilee with Jesus and glimpse a new vision of the meaning of *the Fatherhood of God and the brotherhood of man,* or to stroll with Saint Francis of Assisi or Dr. Albert Schweitzer as they fed the birds and perhaps gain a complete new conception of the phrase, *reverence for life.* If I should meet with men from my native land, I could receive many pointers from wise Benjamin Franklin on how to correct bad habits. If I could sit with the Sage of Monticello as he talked with the students of the University of Virginia on *freedom, the rights of men and the tyranny of the state,* I could gain a deeper understanding of the possibilities and limitations of government. If I could walk with the brooding Abraham Lincoln whose statue sits on my desk and absorb something of his growth from obscurity to greatness and to infinite patience, I would surely be a better man for the experience. If I were lucky I might even walk across the campus of what used to be Washington College, now Washington and Lee University, or look out over the beautiful Shenandoah Valley with that boyhood hero of mine, Robert E. Lee, one of the most flawless characters in American history, and absorb from him something of *duty, honor* and *courage,* and this could be a most exciting prospect and most interesting exit.

While I am still enthralled with this Grecian intellectual future a third door comes into view with a Hindu sign and the one word:

Reincarnation.

To my literal mind this simply means another chance, and I think back how often I have completed a long and difficult project in the past and said, "If I could only start over again I could do it better." So, if the Great Playwright should write another chapter to the saga of humanity and call me back for a repeat performance I would gladly respond.

As I dwell on these various exits I recall a few of the vast changes that have occurred in one lifetime. Darwin's theory of evolution became acceptable and then respectable in spite of laws to prevent us from learning about it. Then a man of this period, one of the great minds of all times, Dr. Albert Einstein, wrote a simple formula—$E = MC^2$—and with his theory of relativity stood the scientific community on its head as completely as Darwin had upset the theological community a few decades earlier. When I look at these and other vast changes that have taken place during my life and the tremendous widening of man's horizons I'm inclined to believe that even the wisest of men are incapable of grasping more than a small segment of the grand design, and I am persuaded that the ultimate design of the Divine Playwright for the future of man may prove more amazing, more wonderful and more glorious than any man has ever conceived.

And so these different doors and the different opinions which lie behind them little concern me because before I existed there was the Great Spirit. From whence I came It resided and whither I go there It will also be waiting. And with the conviction that my body, my mind and my spirit are in harmony with the universe and the Maker of the universe, it is easy to rise and face the day with equanimity because I know I will be walking in His presence, or to turn my face to the pillow and go softly to sleep knowing that whenever and wherever I wake there I will find the Great Spirit of the Carolina mountains and the Judean hills.

CREATING YOUR OWN PROGRAM

It is advisable that you read the following guided exercises as an experience to help you consider other programs you might create. Then I will give you a list of additional generalized and specific phrases from which to choose. Of course all positive phrases are satisfactory if they *feel* good to you.

TEN

Guided Exercises

The exercises in this chapter are best done with a guide—a friend, family member, or loved one, or, if possible, a tape recorder. The other person should read them to you, *slowly,* or you may record them for playing back to yourself. Be sure, when you practice, that you allow adequate time to repeat the phrases and to *feel* the suggestion sensation. Also, before you begin, be certain you have chosen your own special healing phrase. It should be a short (12 words or fewer), positive affirmation of your most important goal. *Focus on the creation of the condition desired.*

These guided exercises are not essential for health, but they do add dimension to the practice of Biogenics. They require 15 to 45 minutes each and may be useful for some special purpose. I suggest that you read the rest of the book straight through and select exercises that appeal to you. Try them at least once and you may wish to incorporate one or more in your continuing daily practice. Before you begin, write out your most important goal, physical, social, financial, or any other, and make your own special healing affirmation, such as, "Every day I become healthier and healthier."

The guided exercises are part of the program taught patients at the Pain Rehabilitation Center in La

Crosse, Wisconsin, and are reproduced from our workbook, *Health* (Copyright 1975, by C. Norman Shealy, M.D.). For specific health or organ phrases see pages 175–177.

PROGRESSIVE RELAXATION

Relaxation of Arms

Pause 10 to 15 seconds between sentences.

Settle back as comfortably as you can. Let yourself relax to the best of your ability. Say and practice—

I clench my right fist; I clench my fist tighter and tighter and study the tension as I do so.

I keep it clenched, then feel the tension in my right hand become loose, and observe the contrast in my feelings.

I let myself go and become more relaxed all over.

Once more I clench my right fist really tight.

I hold it, and notice the tension again.

Now I let go, relax; my fingers straighten out, and I notice the difference once more.

I repeat that with my left fist.

I clench my left fist while the rest of my body relaxes.

I clench that fist tighter and feel the tension.

And now I relax.

Again, I enjoy the contrast.

I repeat that once more: I clench my left fist, tight and tense.

Now I do the opposite of tension—I relax, and feel the difference.

I continue relaxing for a while. [*Pause one minute.*]

I clench both fists tighter and tighter, both fists tense, forearms tense.

I study the sensations and I relax.

I straighten out my fingers and feel that relaxation.

I continue relaxing my hands and forearms more and more. [*Pause one minute.*]

Now I bend my elbows and tense my biceps; I tense them harder and study the tension feelings.

I straighten out my arms; I let them relax and feel that difference again.

I allow the relaxation to deepen.

Once more I tense my biceps; I hold the tension and observe it carefully.

I straighten my arms and relax.

I relax to the best of my ability.

I note my feelings when I tense up and when I relax.

Now I straighten my arms; I straighten them so that I feel more tension in the triceps muscles along the back of my arms.

I stretch my arms and feel that tension.

And now I relax.

I place my arms in a comfortable position.

I allow the relaxation to proceed on its own.

My arms feel comfortably heavy as I allow them to relax in the triceps muscles.

I straighten them.

I feel the tension and I relax.

Now I concentrate on pure relaxation in my arms without any tension.

I allow my arms to be comfortable and allow them to relax further and further.

I continue to relax my arms further.

Even when my arms seem fully relaxed, I go that extra bit further.

I achieve deeper and deeper levels of relaxation. [*Pause one minute.*]

Relaxation of Chest, Stomach, and Lower Back

I relax my entire body to the best of my ability.

I feel that comfortable heaviness that accompanies relaxation.

I breathe easily and freely in and out.

I notice that relaxation increases as I exhale.

As I breathe out I feel more relaxed.

Now I breathe in and fill my lungs.

I inhale deeply and hold my breath.

I study the tension.

I exhale, let the walls of my chest grow loose, and push the air out automatically.

I continue relaxing and breathing freely and gently.

I feel the relaxation and enjoy it.

With the rest of my body as relaxed as possible, I fill my lungs again.

I breathe in deeply and hold it.

I breath out and appreciate the relief.

I breathe normally.

I continue relaxing my chest and let the relaxation spread to my back, shoulders, neck, and arms.

I merely let go, and enjoy the relaxation.

Now I notice my abdominal muscles, my stomach area.

I tighten my stomach muscles, make my abdomen hard.

I notice the tension; and I relax.

I allow the muscles to loosen, and notice the contrast.

I press and tighten my stomach muscles.

I hold the tension and study it, and I relax.

I notice the general well-being that comes with relaxing my abdomen.

Now I draw my abdomen in, pulling the muscles right in, and feel the tension this way.

I relax again.

I let my abdomen out.

I continue breathing normally and easily and feel the gentle massaging action all over my chest and abdomen.

Now I pull my abdomen in again, and hold the tension.

I push out and tense my muscles in that position.

I hold the tension.

Once more I pull in and feel the tension.

Now I relax my abdomen fully.

I let the tension dissolve as my relaxation grows deeper.

Each time I breathe out, I notice the rhythmic relaxation both in my lungs and in my abdomen.

I notice my chest and my abdomen relaxing more and more.

I let go of all contractions anywhere in my body.

I direct my attention to my lower back.

I arch my back, making my lower back quite hollow, and feel the tension along my spine.

I settle down comfortably again relaxing my lower back.

I arch my back up and feel the tensions as I do so.

I keep the rest of my body as relaxed as possible.

I localize the tension throughout my lower back area.

I relax once more, and further, and further.

I relax my lower back; my upper back.

I spread the relaxation to my stomach, chest, shoulders, arms, and face.

These parts are relaxing further, and further, and even further.

Relaxation of Facial Area with Neck, Shoulders, and Upper Back

All my muscles are loose and heavy.

I am quiet and comfortable.

I wrinkle up my forehead.

I wrinkle it tighter.

I stop wrinkling my forehead, relax and smooth it out.

I picture my entire forehead and scalp becoming smoother as the relaxation increases.

I frown and crease my brows and study the tension.

I let go of the tension again.

I smooth out my forehead once more.

I close my eyes tighter and tighter.

I feel the tension.

I relax my eyes.

I keep my eyes closed gently, comfortably, and notice the relaxation.

I clench my jaws, biting my teeth together.

I study the tension throughout my jaws.

I relax my jaws now.

I let my lips part slightly.

I appreciate the relaxation.

I press my tongue hard against the roof of my mouth.

I look for the tension.

I let my tongue return to a comfortable and relaxed position.

I press my lips together.

I press my lips together tighter and tighter.

I relax my lips.

I note the contrast between tension and relaxation.

I feel the relaxation all over my face, all over my forehead and scalp, eyes, jaws, lips, tongue, and throat.

The relaxation progresses further and further.

Now I attend to my neck muscles.

I press my head back as far as it can go and feel the tension in my neck.

I roll it to the right and feel the tension shift.

I roll it to the left.

I straighten my head and bring it forward.

I press my chin against my chest.

I let my head return to a comfortable position, and study the relaxation.

I let the relaxation develop.

I shrug my shoulders again and move them around.

I bring my shoulders up and forward and back.

I feel the tension in my shoulders and in my upper back.

I drop my shoulders once more and relax.

I let the relaxation spread deep into my shoulders, right into my back muscles.

I relax my neck and throat, and my jaws and other facial areas as pure pleasant relaxation takes over and grows deeper ... deeper ... even deeper.

Relaxation of Hips, Thighs, and Calves
Followed by Complete Body Relaxation

I let go of all tensions and relax.

I flex my buttocks and thighs.

I flex my thighs by pressing down my heels as hard as I can.

I relax and note the difference.

I straighten my knees and flex my thigh muscles again.

I hold the tension.

I relax my hips and thighs.

I allow the relaxation to proceed on its own.

I press my feet and toes downward, away from my face.

My calf muscles become tense.

I study that tension.

I relax my feet and calves.

I bend my feet toward my face so that I feel tension along my shins.

I bring my toes right up.

I relax again.

I keep relaxing for a while. [*Pause one minute.*]

I let myself relax further all over.

I relax my feet, ankles, calves and shins, knees, thighs, buttocks, and hips.

I feel the pleasant heaviness of my lower body as I relax still further.

I spread the relaxation to my stomach, waist, lower back.

I let go more and more.

I feel the relaxation all over.

I let it proceed to my upper back, chest, shoulders, and arms and right to the tips of my fingers.

I keep relaxing more and more deeply, making sure that my throat remains relaxed.

I relax my neck and jaws and all my facial muscles.

I keep relaxing my whole body like that.

I let myself relax. [*Pause one minute.*]

Now I become twice as relaxed, merely by taking in a really deep breath and slowly exhaling.

With my eyes closed I am less aware of objects and movements around me.

I breathe in deeply and feel myself becoming heavier.

I take in a long, deep breath and let it out very slowly.

I feel how pleasantly heavy and relaxed I have become.

In a state of perfect relaxation I am unwilling to move a single muscle in my body.

I think about the effort that would be required to raise my right arm.

As I *think* about raising my right arm, I notice tension creeping into my shoulder and arm.

I decide not to lift my arm but to continue relaxing.

I observe the relief and the disappearance of the tension. [*Pause one minute.*]

I am relaxed and comfortable [*Repeat 3 times.*]

I see and feel myself filled with universal love. [*Repeat 3 times.*]

And I will carry this love with me throughout each day.

I reach to attain my highest spiritual goals. [*Repeat 3 times.*]

Each time I practice these exercises, I benefit more and more.

Every day in every way I am becoming healthier and healthier.

Now I repeat over and over my own special healing affirmation. And as I do so I see myself accomplishing my goal. [*Pause 5 minutes.*]

I am further and further relaxed.

I am relaxed and comfortable. [*Wait one minute.*]

As I open my eyes I take another deep, relaxing breath and a big, comfortable stretch, feeling my body filled with loving energy.

GENERAL RELAXATION

Letting Go

Begin by allowing your body to be completely re-laxed. Lean back . . . rest your arms beside you . . . and close your eyes. . . . Keep your eyes closed gently, while you learn to relax and repeat:

I am aware of the feelings in my body at this moment. I notice whether I am warm or cold. . . . I feel the chair (or floor) beneath me. . . . I let my body gradually get heavier.

I take a deep breath and hold it . . . now I let it out slowly. . . . I take another deep breath and hold it. . . . I let it out slowly; I feel the tightness going out of my chest and body. . . . Feelings of deep relaxation are beginning to spread to all parts of my body.

I now focus my attention on my hands; I notice the feelings from them and let go of the muscles; I relax the muscles in my hands . . . even more than I'm doing now. I allow my hands and fingers gradually to become looser and heavier. . . .

I let the relaxation begin to flow from the muscles of my fingers and hands . . . up through my wrists . . . and into my forearms. I feel my forearms getting looser and heavier. . . . I enjoy the pleasant feeling of my hands and forearms, my hands and forearms getting looser and heavier; I let go of my muscles.

I let go now in my upper arms. . . . The relaxation is moving from muscle to muscle . . . a pleasantly heavy feeling is coming into my arms. I am getting more deeply relaxed, heavier . . . more relaxed, heavier, more relaxed. Letting go is voluntary . . . I think of relaxing and I can feel the muscles getting looser and heavier.

Now I let the relaxation move up through my shoulders and into my neck. . . . The pad behind me is completely supporting my head so that my neck muscles can loosen, and I relax. . . . I let the muscles in my neck slacken. . . . I become limp . . . getting more and more relaxed.

I pay attention to my scalp. . . . I smooth out my scalp. . . . I let the muscles become loose and limp. . . . A heavy, relaxed feeling is spreading across my scalp. I smooth out my forehead; I imagine it getting smooth and relaxed. . . . The heavy feeling is flowing down across my face. . . . I relax the muscles around my eyes . . . letting go of the muscles. . . . My eyes remain gently closed. . . . I relax my cheeks. . . . My jaw muscles and the muscles around my mouth are also getting heavier and more relaxed. . . . I feel them gradually becoming heavier and more relaxed . . . growing more deeply relaxed. . . . The relaxation is spreading to my throat.

The relaxation is now flowing down into my chest. . . . I relax my chest. . . . I enjoy the sensation. . . . I feel the muscles of my body gradually getting looser and more relaxed. . . .

I notice now the muscles in my abdomen. . . . I feel these muscles getting looser. . . . I think of letting go of these muscles. . . . I feel these muscles getting looser . . . and more relaxed. . . . Now I relax the muscles in my back, my upper and lower back. . . . All the tightness is leaving my back.

The muscles around my hips and thighs are getting looser and more relaxed. . . . I feel how heavy my body is becoming . . . pressing pleasantly into the chair. . . . I just let myself get heavier . . . gradually get looser . . . and more relaxed. . . . I can feel the wave of relaxation spreading down through my chest, stomach, and hips. . . . The relaxation is deep . . . deeper and deeper . . . heavier and more relaxed. I let the relaxation flow down my legs . . . through my knees . . . now into my calves. . . . I relax my calves. . . . I think of relaxing my calf muscles . . . very deeply relaxed. I relax the muscles in my feet . . . I let my feet get relaxed . . . more and . . . more . . . and more relaxed. . . . My whole body is still growing heavier . . . getting more relaxed.

I tune in to any part of my body where there may still be some tightness. . . . I just think of relaxing those parts, and I find that they become much more relaxed than they now are. . . . I continue relaxing. I enjoy it. . . . I let myself sink deeper and heavier into relaxation. I spend a few minutes enjoying the feeling of deep relaxation that has spread to all parts of my body. [*Pause 2 minutes.*]

I am relaxed and comfortable. [*3 times*]

I see and feel myself filled with universal love and I will carry this love with me throughout each day. [*3 times.*]

I am in tune with my highest spiritual goals. [*3 times*]

Each time I practice these exercises, I benefit more and more.

Every day in every way I am becoming healthier and healthier.

Now I repeat over and over my own special healing affirmation. As I do so, I see myself accomplishing my goal.

I relax deeper and deeper; I am relaxed and comfortable. [*Wait one minute.*] As I open my eyes, I take another deep, relaxing breath and a big, comfortable stretch, feeling the energy flowing throughout my body.

Variations on a Theme

While I talk I would like you to get yourself as
comfortable as you can. . . . Let your eyes close
gently. . . . Listen to my words. . . . Make sure
you're comfortable. It's all right to change position
during the session if you want to . . . or you can
lie relaxed just as you are now. Repeat after me:
I am aware of the feelings in my body at this
moment. . . . I notice whether I am warm or cold.
I feel the chair or mattress beneath me. . . . I let
my body gradually get heavier.

I think of my *left hand*. . . . I just tune in on my
left hand. . . . I pay attention to the feelings from
it and let go of the muscles in it. . . . I let go of the
muscles in my left hand even more, . . . allowing
it gradually to become looser and heavier. . . .

Now my *right hand* . . . I think of my right hand
getting looser . . . heavier . . . just letting go . . .
of the muscles in my right hand . . . letting go
further . . . more deeply. . . . And now I feel the
relaxation coming into my left and right *forearms*. . . . I feel my forearms getting looser
and heavier. . . . I enjoy the relaxation that is now
coming into my forearms. . . . My hands and forearms are getting looser and heavier. . . . I let go
of my muscles.

I am letting go now in my *upper arms* . . . both
my left and right upper arms . . . getting more
deeply relaxed . . . getting heavier, more relaxed
. . . deeper and deeper. . . . As I continue to think
of letting go of my muscles I am able to make
them even looser and more relaxed than they are
now. Anywhere I can feel any tension in my left
or right hands and arms, I just let go of the tensions as I did before. . . . Letting go is voluntary
. . . pleasantly under my control. As I think of letting go I can feel each muscle getting looser and

heavier. . . . I am letting go now in my *shoulders* . . . both my left and my right shoulders . . . are getting very heavy now . . . heavier and heavier . . . getting as loose and relaxed as my hands and arms . . . getting still more relaxed . . . more and more relaxed. . . .

Now I pay attention to my *forehead*. . . . I smooth out my forehead. . . . I just imagine it getting smoothed and relaxed. . . . I let go of the muscles . . . and the muscles around my *eyes*. . . . My eyes remain gently closed. It's easy to lie here letting go of all my muscles and enjoying the feelings that accompany this deep muscle relaxation.

Now I pay attention to my *cheeks*. . . . As my cheeks get very comfortable . . . relaxed . . . I think of the muscles beneath my eyes and my cheeks get looser and more relaxed. . . . My *jaw* muscles and the muscles around my *mouth* are also getting heavier and more relaxed. . . . I continue to let go of all my muscles . . . feeling them gradually becoming heavier and more relaxed . . . growing more deeply relaxed . . . the relaxation spreading on to my *neck*. . . .

I notice the feelings in my *chest* . . . and continue to enjoy the sensation. . . . Letting go of my muscles is a voluntary thing which I am learning to bring under my own regulation . . . and I can feel myself gradually getting looser and more relaxed. . . . I pay attention now to the muscles in my *abdomen*. I feel the muscles getting looser. . . . I think of letting go of these muscles. . . . I feel them gradually getting heavier . . . more deeply relaxed . . . still further relaxed. . . . My muscles are getting looser. . . . The muscles around my *hips* and *thighs* are getting looser and more relaxed. . . . I feel how pleasantly heavy my body is becoming. . . . It even feels that it is pressing down into the chair or mattress . . . getting heavier. . . . I let myself become heavier. . . . I let my muscles go . . . gradually get looser . . . and more relaxed. I can feel the wave of relaxation spreading down my forehead, through my face, and my neck, through my chest, stomach and hips . . . coming now into my thighs. My thighs now sharing the deep relaxation . . . deeper and deeper . . . heavier and more relaxed . . . I let my *calves* get more relaxed.

I think of relaxing my calf muscles . . . letting them get heavier and looser . . . very deeply relaxed. . . . I relax now the muscles in my *feet*. . . . I let my feet get relaxed . . . more . . . and more relaxed . . . my whole body still growing heavier . . . getting more relaxed. . . .

I notice now any place in my body that may still be a little bit tense. . . . I tune in anywhere where there may still be some tension. . . . If there are no tensions left I continue relaxing . . . but if there are, I think of relaxing those parts. And if I still feel tension anywhere . . . I temporarily tighten up that muscle . . . and let go of it the way I did before. [*Pause one minute.*] I continue relaxing . . . but if I still have some tensions anywhere . . . I take care of them either by letting go of the muscles or by first tensing them and then letting them go. . . . I continue relaxing as I have been. . . . I let myself get heavier and sink deeper into the chair (or mattress) . . . heavier and deeper. . . . I notice the pleasant feelings of warmth that come into my body as I get more and more deeply relaxed . . . comfortably relaxed. . . . I am aware of a tingling sensation in my *fingertips* and my *toes*. . . . All these sensations are perfectly natural consequences of relaxing my muscles very deeply . . . growing deeper . . . and still deeper . . . getting heavier and more relaxed. . . . I just let myself get more deeply relaxed. . . . As I think of letting go even more, my muscles will naturally become looser . . . and looser . . . and heavy . . . and relaxed . . . deeply and comfortably relaxed. . . . [*Pause one minute.*]

I am relaxed and comfortable. [*3 times*]

I reach to attain my highest spiritual goals. [*3 times*]

I see and feel myself filled with universal love. [*3 times*]

I will carry that love with me throughout each day. Each time I practice these exercises, I benefit more and more. Every day in every way I am becoming healthier and healthier.

Now I repeat over and over my own special healing affirmation. And as I do so I see myself accomplishing my goal. [*Pause 5 minutes.*]

I am relaxed and comfortable. [*4 times*] [*Pause one minute.*] As I open my eyes I take another deep, relaxing breath and a big comfortable stretch, feeling my body filled with loving energy.

Developing Calm and Serenity

Begin by getting as comfortable as you can. Settle back comfortably. Just try to let go of all the tension in your body. Now take in a deep breath. Breathe right in and hold it. And now exhale. Just let the air out quite automatically and feel a calmer feeling beginning to develop. Now just carry on breathing normally and just concentrate on feeling heavy all over in a pleasant way. Study your own body heaviness. This should give you a calm and reassuring feeling all over. Now work on tension and relaxation. Repeat and do these activities.

I tense every muscle in my body, every muscle: my jaws. I tighten my eyes, my shoulder muscles, my arms, chest, back, stomach, legs, every part just tensing and tensing. I feel the tension all over my body—tighter and tighter—tensing everywhere, and now I let it go, just stop tensing and relax. I feel a wave of calm that comes over me as I stop tensing like that. A definite wave of calm.

I notice the contrast between the slight tensions that are there when my eyes are open and the dis-

appearance of those surface tensions as I close
my eyes. So, while relaxing the rest of my body, I
open my eyes and feel the surface tensions which
will disappear when I close my eyes. I close my
eyes and feel the greater degree of relaxation with
my eyes closed. I keep my eyes closed and take a
deep, deep breath and hold it. I relax the rest of
my body as well as I can and notice the tension
from holding my breath. I study the tension. I let
out my breath and feel the deepening relaxation. I
go with it, beautifully relaxing now. I breathe normally and feel the relaxation flowing into my forehead and scalp. I think of each part as I feel it
—relaxing—just letting go, easing up, eyes and
nose, facial muscles. I feel a tingling sensation as
the relaxation flows in. I feel a warm sensation. I
enjoy the relaxation now spreading very beautifully
into my face, into lips, jaws, tongue, and mouth
so that my lips are slightly parted as my jaw
muscles relax further and further. My throat and
neck are relaxing and my shoulder and upper back
are relaxing, further and further. I feel the relaxation flowing into my arms and to the very tips of
my fingers. I feel the relaxation in my chest as I
breathe regularly and easily. The relaxation is
flowing down even under my armpits and down
my sides, right into my abdomen. The relaxation
of my abdomen and lower back spreads all the
way through in a warm, penetrating way, calm,
and down my hips, buttocks, and thighs to the
very tips of my toes. The waves of relaxation just
travel down my calves to my ankles and toes. I feel
relaxed from head to toe. Each time I practice this
I find a deeper level of relaxation being achieved
—a deeper serenity and calm, a good feeling.

Now to increase the feelings of relaxation at this
point, each time I exhale, each time I breathe out
for the next minute, I think the word "relax." I
think the word "relax" as I breathe out. [*Pause
one minute.*] I feel that deeper relaxation and
carry on relaxing. I feel a deeper, deeper feeling of

relaxation. To further increase the benefits, I feel the emotional calm, those tranquil and serene feelings which embrace me all over inside and out, a feeling of safe security, a calm indifference. Those are the feelings that relaxation enables me to capture more and more effectively each time I practice a relaxation sequence. Relaxation allows me to feel a quiet inner confidence—a good feeling about myself. Now once more I feel the heavy sensations that accompany relaxation as my muscles switch off so that I feel in good contact with my environment, nicely together, the heavy, good feeling of calm and security, tranquillity and serenity.

Now I deepen the relaxation still further by just using some very special stimulus words. I use words *calm* and *serene*. I repeat calm and serene for one minute. [*Pause one minute.*] I feel the deepening—ever, ever deepening—waves of relaxation as I feel so much more calm and serene. I think of the words and feel the sensations over and over.

I am relaxed and comfortable. [*3 times*]

I reach to attain my highest spiritual goals. [*3 times*]

I see and feel myself filled with universal love. [*3 times*]

And I will carry this love with me throughout each day. Each time I practice these exercises, I benefit more and more. Every day in every way I am becoming healthier and healthier.

Now I repeat over and over my own personal healing phrase. As I say my healing affirmation I see myself accomplishing my goal. [*Pause 5 minutes.*]

I breathe deeply and completely. [*4 times*] [*Pause one minute.*] As I open my eyes I take another

deep, relaxing breath and a big comfortable
stretch, feeling myself filled with loving energy.

PHYSIOLOGICAL EXERCISE

[Speak slowly. Pause 15 seconds after each body
area.]

The reason that you start Biogenics exercises with
deep breathing is that normally, as I've said, you
have both voluntary and involuntary (or automatic) regulation of respiration. So, just for a
moment, notice your respiration. Breathe deeply
in and deeply out, deeper and deeper into relaxation, more and more relaxed, breathing deeply and
comfortably; feel the air moving in, feel the air
moving out. Don't go to sleep now! Practice the
exercise, practice the feeling. And repeat to yourself each sentence: I concentrate all my mental energy on my scalp. I allow only the sensations from
my scalp to come to my awareness. I hear only the
sound of these words. I block out all other sounds.
I block all sensations except those from my scalp
and allow the feelings from my scalp to come in
pleasantly. I may feel itchy, I may feel tingly.
Whatever I feel within my scalp is a sensation
coming from my body.* My scalp begins to turn
warm. And having achieved the sensation of
warmth within my scalp, I tell my scalp to relax.

I then examine the parts of my face. I allow just
for a few moments the natural sensations that
come from my face to have their say. I allow them
time to speak to me. I feel my forehead. I feel my
eyes. I feel my nose and cheeks. I am aware of my
lips and chin. I feel my ears, and in my entire face
I reach beyond all the normal superficial sensations and feel my heart beating gently, pulsating,
carrying food, oxygen, and warmth throughout my

---

*NOTE: Any focusing of attention on the heartbeat within the scalp
has been deliberately avoided, as patients with migraine should *never*
allow that pulsating sensation in the skull or scalp to become conscious.

face. And as my face becomes warm, I tell it that I appreciate it, for all that it does for me, for responding to me in this way, and I tell it, relax, relax.

I concentrate all my mental energy now on my neck and throat. I feel my neck and throat— no other sensation except those coming from my neck and throat. Fullness, tension, whatever there may be, I allow them to come in; I feel my neck. I don't move it; I just feel it and reach deep within my neck to feel my heart beating. I feel the gentle, calm, regular pulsations of my heartbeat in my neck and throat; and as I do so, I feel my neck and throat becoming warm.

Mentally, with my mind's eye, I reach down and touch my shoulders, arms, forearms, hands, and fingers. I feel all the parts of my arms and as I feel my arms, I feel my heart beating gently and calmly throughout my fingertips, hands, and arms and feel them turn warm. I am thankful for all the great things that they do for me and I tell them, relax.

I am aware of my chest, no other part of my body; I am just aware of my chest. I am aware of my skin, breasts, muscles, rib cage. I am aware of my lungs. I feel them doing their job as my body breathes itself, calmly, gently, and completely. I feel the oxygen coming in. I feel the tension going out, the carbon dioxide going out, and I feel my heart beating. That great magnificent organ that does such a splendid job in distributing blood, oxygen, and food. I feel my heart beat. I am aware of it. I am appreciative of the job that it does, beating 60 times or more every minute, every hour, every day throughout the year and I tell my chest, thank you. Relax, relax.

I feel my abdomen. There are a great many organs within my abdomen, more big important organs than in any other part of my body. I feel them. I examine them. I am aware of their sensations. I allow them each to have their say. I feel my stomach. Coming off the bottom of my stomach, I feel my small intestines wrapping their way around the pancreas. I feel my pancreas and feel my small intestines going down into my colon and rectum. I feel my intestines. Coming back up into the upper abdomen, I feel on the right side my liver and gallbladder. I am aware of my liver. All kinds of chemical activities are going on there. Such an important factory.

And in my left upper abdomen, I feel my spleen, of vital importance in my immune mechanism and in clotting mechanisms. Just beneath my liver and my spleen on either side, I feel my kidneys and riding up on top of my kidneys, my adrenal glands. I feel them. I appreciate their great job producing cortisone, adrenalin, and other important hormones. I feel my kidneys, think about their job, am aware of the filtering they do, taking out excess water and excess salt and chemicals of various sorts, including products of the nitrogen breakdown. And the little tubes leading from my kidneys down into my bladder, my ureters. I am aware of them. I can feel them as I visualize them in my mind's eye and my bladder itself.

I am aware of my pelvic organs and my sex organs. And I appreciate the joy they bring. I am aware of them, feel them.

And, throughout my entire abdomen, my aorta is carrying blood, pulsating strongly, but gently, calmly, and regularly, carrying warmth to all parts of my abdomen and especially to my solar plexus, that great network of nerves of the autonomic nervous system through which I can help control the balance of function in all these organs. I am thankful for my aorta, for my solar plexus, and all those remarkable organs within my abdomen. I feel my heart beating there. I feel my abdomen become warm and tell my abdomen, relax, relax.

This is an exercise which is so important I take my time concentrating on each part of my body as I go through it.

I feel my back, from my neck down to my tailbone. I feel my back, skin, muscles, bones, joints, nerves, spinal cord—I feel them all. All kinds of interesting and good sensations coming from my back. I feel my back turning warm as I feel the pulsations of my heartbeat there.

I feel my buttocks and hips. I let every sensation come in from that great mass of muscles across my buttocks. What a terrific job they do in allowing me to sit. I feel my buttocks. But I also reach deep within and feel my heart beating. I search until I feel the pulsations of my heartbeat within my buttocks and as I do so, I feel my buttocks turn warm and tell them to relax.

I feel the upper parts of my legs, my thighs, the longest and biggest muscles of my body. Huge groups of muscles surrounding one long bone, my femur. I feel those parts of my anatomy. I don't move them; I just feel them; and I feel my heart beating within my thighs, pulsating, carrying the blood, oxygen, and food. I feel my thighs turning warm and tell them to relax.

I feel my knees, great big joints, second in size only to my hip joints. I feel my knees. I am aware of them. I am aware of my throbbing, pulsing heartbeat transmitting blood, food and oxygen, and warmth into my knees and I tell them, relax. I am aware of my calves. They add the spring to my walk and gait. Nice big muscles behind and solid bone out front. I feel my lower legs and calves and especially feel the warmth delivered to my calves by my heartbeat.

I feel my ankles, feet, and toes. I feel them. I appreciate them especially and feel my heart beating gently and calmly within the various parts of my feet and toes and feel them turning warm;

and I tell my feet to relax. Thank you, this is your chance to relax.

These are the physiological ways in which I feel the sensations that are necessary for tuning into my autonomic nervous system. I go through these exercises, enjoying the sensations, comfortable and relaxed, appreciating what is happening, appreciating the ability of my body to respond to my communication. I allow my body to relax indirectly by relaxing my autonomic nervous system in each part of my body. I have relaxed all parts of my body except my brain and mind. That is where it all originates. That is where all those sensations are allowed to come into my consciousness. I go within my mind now and concentrate more on what is important to my mind. I know that to put my mind at rest, I must get rid of all the negative thoughts and activities that go on within my mind; so, I say to myself as I look within, "Okay, I don't have any need for those things anymore. They haven't helped me, so I release them. But not for anyone else to have them—I release them into the care of God. I release all my negative feelings and emotions, all anger, all frustration, all fear, all sadness, all guilt, all depression. I release all my human relations, all the problems that go with them, and my past which is completed. I release my past. And the present, which is here and upon me. I release it and the future. I can plan and make changes in it if I like, but I release the future to be as it will."

And when I have released all these negative things and relaxed all my body and my mind, then I forgive all others their faults and I forgive myself. I reach for my highest loving self. That is the true me. I am attuned to my most loving self. I fill myself with the golden light of love, joy, happiness, peace. I focus my awareness on love and peace. I can focus this way any time I want by thinking only in terms of relaxation and peace and happiness, joy and love. Any time I want, any time there is a problem, I know that I can come back in tune with myself by placing myself in this state of body and mind, so that my body and mind are working lovingly together. It is such a joy to feel this way, to see and feel only light and joy and happiness and love. That's what I would like, that is what I want to feel—only light, joy, and love.

I continue resting in this state allowing myself to be perfectly attuned with love. My body continues its functions normally, breathing easily and comfortably, my heartbeat is calm and regular. All the parts of my body are warm, pulsating gently, happy, relaxed. [*Pause one minute.*]

Now, very, very slowly, very, very slowly, I become aware again of all the things outside my body; gently, slowly, I take a deep breath, I open my eyes and look around feeling comfortable, relaxed, joyful. I take a big, comfortable stretch, feeling myself filled with perfect, loving energy.

IDEAL RELAXATION

This is a technique for ideal, perfect relaxation. First of all, find yourself the most comfortable position possible. Do not cross your arms and legs. Close your eyes. Take a deep, pleasant, comfortable breath, slowly, and let it all out. Relax.

All the parts of your body and mind are now going to work together to achieve perfect, complete relaxation. Allow each muscle in your entire body to go limp and loose, completely relaxed. Feel the tension draining out of your feet and your legs and now you yourself are stating these feelings mentally to yourself: I feel my legs relaxing. All the muscle tension is draining out of my legs. My abdomen is relaxing more and more. My chest is pleasantly, comfortably relaxed. My shoulders, arms, and hands are limp and comfortably relaxed. My neck is totally relaxed. All the parts of my face are totally, completely relaxed. I feel only muscle relaxation in every part of my body.

My arms and legs are heavy and warm. [*3 times*]

My heartbeat is calm and regular. [*3 times*]

My body breathes itself freely and comfortably. [*3 times*]

My abdomen is warm. [*3 times*]

My forehead is cool. [*3 times*]

My mind is quiet and still. [*3 times*]

I am at peace.

I am totally, completely relaxed and comfortable.

And in my mind's eye, I am creating a vision of the most perfect, beautiful, natural area of relaxation that I can posssibly conceive. I see my own ideal spot of relaxation, the one area in all the world where I am happiest, most comfortable, most relaxed, my own ideal spot of relaxation. I see it, feel it, smell it, hear it, taste it. I project myself into my ideal place of relaxation, and as I see myself moving into my ideal area, I see and feel my entire body becoming normal, functioning completely, healthfully, comfortably.

All the parts of my body, mind, and emotions are functioning ideally. I see and feel my body and mind working in complete, perfect harmony. My mind is alert and very, very clear. My vision is bright and distinct. My hearing is excellent. My sensations of taste and smell are functioning pleasantly, normally. My neck is comfortable, flexible, and strong. My thyroid gland balances my metabolism perfectly. My shoulders, arms, and hands are strong and well coordinated.

All the parts of my chest are functioning perfectly. My lungs are bringing in all the oxygen I need, freely, comfortably. They are carrying away all the carbon dioxide. My heartbeat is calm and regular, strongly carrying to all the parts of my body blood, food, oxygen, and warmth.

All my blood chemistries are perfectly balanced and normal. My blood count is healthy and normal. My blood sugar, calcium, all the salts within my blood are in normal, perfect balance. My blood pressure is at a steady, normal level. My immune system is functioning perfectly to protect me from all infections and cancer.

My stomach is digesting my food with ease; and the digestive process is completed comfortably and pleasantly in my small intestine. My colon is absorbing food and water and carrying away the surplus. My pancreas is functioning in a perfectly normal fashion. It produces digestive enzymes and insulin for perfect, normal regulation of my blood sugar. My liver is producing bile to help digestion and is manufacturing all the proper proteins, fats, carbohydrates, and enzymes that are needed throughout my body.

My spleen is helping to regulate my blood-clotting mechanism and my immune system perfectly. My adrenal glands are balancing my blood pressure and all my blood salts and producing a normal amount of adrenalin and cortisone. My kidneys are filtering my blood perfectly, taking out surplus salts and water and transporting them down through the ureters into my bladder which is comfortably reserving them until it is adequately filled with urine. All my pelvic and sex organs are functioning comfortably and pleasantly. My spine is flexible and strong. My legs are strong and well coordinated.

All the parts of my body, mind, emotions, and spirit are functioning harmoniously. I see and feel myself functioning normally, totally, perfectly, in every possible way. In this state of body and mind,

I remain in my ideal place of relaxation, comfortable, relaxed, happy. I am attuned to my purest highest loving self. I see myself filled with and surrounded by love. Only universal love may enter.

Now I repeat over and over my own personal healing affirmation. As I do so I see myself accomplishing my goal. [*Pause 5 minutes.*]

Now I take a deep, pleasant, comfortably relaxing breath and relax even further in the knowledge that I am creating in my body and mind the healthy feelings and images that I have been seeing. And I will carry these back with me to my normal level of awareness. By focusing my consciousness in this way, I am helping my body, mind, and spirit to achieve my own ideal goals. Every day in every way I am becoming healthier and healthier. I take a deep breath, slowly open my eyes, and take a big stretch. I look around, feeling fine, feeling refreshed and rejuvenated and carrying with me the knowledge that my body and mind are functioning perfectly, healthfully.

COMBINATION EXERCISE

This is a technique for inducing very deep relaxation by combining phrases from several different exercises.

[*Pause 10 seconds after each sentence.*]

Do this exercise lying on your back, your legs out straight and uncrossed, your arms comfortable, either folded acrosss your abdomen or beside you.

You may have a pillow beneath your knees; you may have a small pillow under your head.

Assume the position that is most tolerable and comfortable.

Close your eyes.

Take three deep, slow breaths and repeat silently
to yourself: Now I am going to instruct my body
and mind in techniques for relaxation.

First, I think about my right hand and arm and
allow them to become heavy and warm.

My right arm is heavy and warm and relaxed and
comfortable.

I allow this sensation to spread across my shoulders to my left arm and hand.

My left arm and hand are becoming heavy and
warm.

My left arm and hand are heavy and warm.

My left arm and hand are heavy and warm and
relaxed and comfortable.

I allow the sensation to flow down my back and
legs.

My legs are becoming heavy and warm and relaxed.

My legs are heavy and warm and relaxed.

My legs are heavy and warm and relaxed and
comfortable.

I allow this sensation to flow up into my abdomen
and in the solar plexus area.

My abdomen and all its contents are becoming
heavy and relaxed.

My abdomen and solar plexus are heavy and relaxed and warm.

My abdomen and solar plexus are heavy and
warm, relaxed and comfortable.

My whole body is heavy and warm.

My body is heavy and warm and relaxed and
comfortable.

In this state, I am so comfortable and so relaxed that I do not have to work to control my breathing; my body breathes itself, freely and comfortably.

My body breathes itself.

My body breathes itself.

My body is heavy and warm, relaxed and comfortable, and it breathes itself.

In this state of relaxation and automatic breathing, my heartbeat is regular.

My heartbeat is calm and regular.

My heartbeat is calm and regular.

My heartbeat is calm and regular.

My body is in tune with my mind and spirit.

My body and mind are relaxed and warm and comfortable.

My body and mind are relaxed, warm, comfortable, and happy.

All about me is happy, relaxed, and comfortable.

I am perfectly in harmony with my body, mind, and spirit.

All are relaxed, warm and comfortable and happy.

In this state of heavy relaxation, warmth and comfort, I allow my body to begin to expand.

Instead of being a heavy relaxation, it becomes a light, airy relaxation starting down at my feet.

I imagine that my feet are expanding in all directions by one inch, pulsating and growing with each breath and each heartbeat.

One inch bigger.

I allow this one-inch expansion to spread up into my legs and around my knees.

Up into my thighs expanding by one inch and on up into my lower abdomen and around my back, expanding comfortably by one inch in all directions.

I allow this to continue on up into my upper back and around into my chest, expanding by one inch in all directions.

Now, into my shoulders, down into my arms, hands, and fingers, expanding by one inch, comfortably.

Up over my neck and around my head, expanding by one inch.

Starting back down at my feet, I allow myself to expand by twelve inches in all directions, expansion comfortably pulsating twelve inches around my feet and toes and up over my ankles, expanding comfortably in all directions.

And this expansion is going up around the calves and knees into my thighs, twelve inches of relaxed, pulsating, expanded body and mind; comfortable and relaxed.

The expansion flows into my lower abdomen and around my back, comfortable, warm and expanded.

I allow myself to continue feeling this expansion spread into my upper chest, front and back, and across my shoulders, expanding by twelve inches, over my arms and hands and fingers all expanded by twelve inches and up my neck and around my head so that my entire body, mind and soul, all are expanded by twelve inches, comfortably, happily, warm.

I am light and relaxed, warm and comfortable and happy.

I am in tune with myself and with the universe.

My whole body with each pulsation of my heart-beat, with every breath, is becoming more relaxed, more expanded, and more comfortable than it has ever been before.

I relax and enjoy this comfort, this expansion.

I continue pulsating, growing, and expanding.

I am expanded and comfortable, pulsating, relaxed, warm, comfortable and happy.

Every day in every way I am becoming more and more healthy and happy.

My body and mind are working together as one with nature, with the universe, with God.

The universal life force of love is within me.

I am comfortable, happy, expanded, and relaxed.

I am so relaxed and expanded and comfortable that my body feels as if it were floating.

I reach down *mentally* and feel my lovely expanded, comfortable, warm, pulsating feet and they feel as light and fluffy as one of the clouds floating by.

And as I reach up my body, mentally caressing it, it is as if I were being caressed by a warm summer breeze.

My whole body is relaxed and expanded, comfortable, warm, and I feel a great joy and happiness in this relaxation and expansion.

My whole body is relaxed, comfortable, and expanded.

I am at peace with myself and with the world.

My body remains expanded, relaxed, and comfortable, and always my hands, feet, legs and arms, and knees and elbows are expanded, relaxed and comfortable.

I am free of pains and worries.

My chest, heart, abdomen, stomach and intestines, spleen, liver, kidneys, all my hormone glands are relaxed, expanded, comfortable, warm, and happy.

Most of all, my mind and soul are expanded, warm, comfortable, and happy.

I forgive myself for all past problems.

I forgive all those around me.

I feel only love.

The world is a part of me and I am a part of it.

Nature and the universe are expanded and comfortable.

I am free of pain; I feel only relaxation, expansion, pulsation.

I am free of pain in every part of my body; I am comfortable.

I feel only joy and happiness, expansion and relaxation, warmth and comfort.

My entire body is comfortable, warm, expanded.

I understand and forgive all problems in myself and others.

I am expanded, comfortable, in tune with myself.

My heartbeat is calm and regular.

My body breathes itself.

My muscles and nerves and all of the parts of my body are relaxed and comfortable and expanded.

I am relaxed and comfortable. [*3 times*]

I reach to attain my highest spiritual self. [*3 times*]

I see and feel myself filled with universal love. [*3 times*]

And I will carry this love with me throughout each day.

Each time I practice these exercises, I benefit more and more.

Every day in every way I am becoming healthier and healthier.

Now I repeat over and over my own special healing affirmation. As I do so I see myself accomplishing my goal. [*Pause 5 minutes.*]

I breathe deeply and completely. [*4 times*] [*Wait one minute.*]

As I open my eyes I take another deep relaxing breath and a big comfortable stretch, feeling myself filled with perfect loving energy.

SQUIRMING; HAND LEVITATION

This exercise requires one hour and includes a variety of experiences.

One of the techniques, which is very easy to do and which we all need every day, sometimes many times a day, is squirming. We all squirm to adjust our body's discomforts. So, we are now going to squirm—purposefully.

If you are lying too close to another person or object so that when you shake and squirm you are going to hit something, move out a little before we start. You can squirm sitting up. You know we all do it; you shift your weight around. You can squirm standing up, any way you like. But lying down is probably the easiest way to relax your body and your mind by squirming. So, before we start, kick, stretch, get everything out there so you know you have room to squirm. This is a physical technique for relaxing.

OK, now, first of all, take a deep breath, close your eyes, be visually unaware of the activities around you. Be unaware of sound except for what I say, and repeat that to yourself as you visualize.

I imagine that my entire body is surrounded by a big, loose, red balloon, and I am going to stretch out and squirm around and stretch that big balloon in all directions, just really wiggle, and push it out away from me and stretch it in all directions. *Squirm!* I stretch that red balloon out as big as it can be. I take a deep breath and relax. [*Pause.*]

I imagine that I am now within a big orange balloon and I am going to stretch that orange balloon in all directions; so I wiggle my body and stretch out in all directions and kick and hit and squirm around until I have that balloon stretched as far as it can go. *Squirm!* I take a deep breath and relax. [*Pause.*]

I imagine that I am within a great big yellow balloon and reach out again and *squirm!* I kick and hit and strike and stretch that yellow balloon in all directions as far as I can. I take a deep breath and relax. [*Pause.*]

I imagine that I am in a great big green balloon and reach out and kick and squirm. I stretch out that green balloon in all directions in every way I can and when that green balloon is nicely stretched, I take another deep breath and relax. [*Pause.*]

I imagine that I am in a blue balloon and as I come into that blue balloon, I reach out again and *squirm.* I stretch and kick and expand that blue balloon in all directions, big as it can go. I take another deep breath and relax. [*Pause.*]

I imagine that I am now in a lovely white balloon, brilliant and pure white, and I stretch out in all directions and *squirm.* I kick and stretch that white balloon until it is as big as it will go. I take a deep breath and relax. [*Pause.*]

I feel so good being in this big, comfortable, white balloon that I would just like to spread it out over the whole world, so I reach out with my hand and pick up a sharp needle. And I take that needle and thrust it into the side of my white balloon. It breaks and spreads all over the world. I relax. [*Pause.*]

I breathe deeply and comfortably. I allow my body and mind to float with this balloon throughout the world, spreading light and joy in all directions. I picture myself going with this great balloon of whiteness, joy, and love everywhere, and I breathe deeply and comfortably. I allow my body to breathe itself. My heartbeat is calm and regular. I take a deep, deep breath and relax. All parts of my body and mind are now relaxed and in tune with one another, at peace and at rest; I am relaxed.

I allow my neck to go loose. I move my head from side to side and round about in a circle one way and then the other and then I reverse the movement again and then I relax my neck and lie back flat and comfortable. [*Pause.*]

I raise my right foot about twelve inches up in the air and stiffen out all the muscles in my leg and make it as tight and stiff as I can so that it gets tired and I begin thinking of the muscles. I think about them, tight, tense, firmly contracted, tense as they can be; my eyes are closed, and I see those tight muscles in my mind's eye, and while I am tensely contracting those muscles in my right leg, I can't possibly remember my neck muscles and my shoulders and they have to be relaxed; and when my leg becomes so tired that I can't do anything more with it, I let it drop back down to the floor *heavily*, limp.

And as soon as it falls down, I raise up my left leg and make my left leg tense, tight; I strain every muscle within my left leg and again mentally follow the tight muscles from my toe to my hip; I feel each muscle from my toes all the way up to my hip joint tighten up and be as tight as they can be and then my leg becomes really tired. I let my left leg drop quickly back down to the floor.

I then raise my right arm up in the air, stiff as a board, stiff and tight, and clench my fist straight up over my body. I stiffen and tighten my muscles as much as I can. I let every muscle feel tight as a steel band and follow in my thoughts each muscle from my fingertips up to my shoulder and neck. It will take a longer time for my arm to tire than it did for my legs, but I just keep them there, tense as can be. I forget every other part of my body because I am really concentrating on making my arm stiff and tight. Every muscle in there is tense as a board, fully contracted. But, when it gets tired, I let it fall back down beside me.

And immediately, I raise my left arm up, stiff as a board, tight as can be and hold it there and mentally squeeze my fingers tight and clench like a boxer, tensing my arm as if I were going into battle and thinking only of keeping it up there until it is really tired, totally exhausted, and I let it fall back down beside me.

And when it has, I then stiffen out my whole body, all my back and my chest and my abdomen and really stiffen out, tight, tight, every muscle within me; but I don't forget to breathe. When I feel as though my body is totally stiff and tight and tired, I let it go loose and relax and take a deep breath. [*Pause.*]

I keep my eyes closed, but I imagine on the ceiling above me a circle four feet in diameter, and I allow my eyes to move around that circle, starting at one point and, going clockwise, moving completely around it. Then, I reverse direction and go counterclockwise all the way around the circle. And then, my eyes still closed, I visualize on the ceiling above me a square, four feet across, and as I see the square, I start in one corner and move my eyes clockwise all the way around the square; and then, going counterclockwise, I move my eyes around the square. Then I catch my eyes and squeeze my eyelids as tightly as they can go; very, very tight, tighter than I thought possible; and I relax them. [*Pause.*]

I take a deep, relaxing breath and release it. I slowly breathe in and out, all parts of my body totally, blissfully relaxed. I relax, breathe slowly again, and now I raise one hand up to my face, fingers a little bit together with my thumb stuck out. I press my thumb against my right nostril, closing it off, leaving my left nostril open. I take a deep, full, and comfortable breath through my left nostril; then I blow it all out. I keep my right nostril closed and take another deep, slow breath and hold it in, hold it while I count 1–2–3–4–5– 6–7–8, and I move my hand to the other side of my nose and with my fingers I enclose my left nostril and breathe out—all the way out. I leave my right nostril open and slowly breathe in through my right nostril keeping my left one closed. I breathe all the way in now and hold it in while I count 1–2–3–4–5–6–7–8, and I quickly shift my hand to the other side and breathe out through my left nostril. Again, I keep my right nostril closed as I take a full breath through my left nostril, 1–2–3–4–5–6–7–8; I close my left nostril and breathe out through my right nostril. I put my fingers on my left nostril and close it. I keep doing this, closing one nostril, breathe in through the other one, hold my breath, then clos- ing the first nostril and breathing out through the opposite one. I breathe in one side and out the other, slowly, comfortably. When I have done that four times, I put my hand back down at my side and continue to breathe deeply and comfortably and slowly. [*Pause 2 minutes.*]

Now I am becoming deeply relaxed. I take a few more deep, comfortable, and easy breaths, concentrating fully upon the sensation as the air enters my lungs and as it goes out; and I allow my body to become more and more relaxed, deeper and deeper and more and more comfortable, more parts of my body increasingly relaxed and more relaxed than I have ever been at any time in my entire life, concentrating only on total, perfect, and blissful relaxation. I am more and more relaxed, more and more comfortable. All parts of my body are fully, pleasantly relaxed; I am concentrating only upon what I am feeling, only the sensation of relaxation as I become more and more deeply relaxed, more and more comfortable. It is a very pleasant sensation, to relax totally and comfortably. I allow my whole body and my mind to be totally at peace and relaxed, very light and very comfortable, more and more relaxed and I will count from 20 down to one and as I do so, I become more and more relaxed. Each time that I count I find myself relaxing more than I did before, deeper and deeper and more and more comfortable, more and more relaxed, more and more pleasant, deeper and deeper and more and more comfortable. Now I count mentally 20–19– relaxing more and more, deeper and deeper and more and more comfortable –18–17–16– deeper and more comfortably relaxed –15– deeper and deeper –14–13–12–11– more relaxed than I have ever been. Each time I practice I am more relaxed than I was the last time, more comfortable, deeper and deeper relaxed –10–9–8–7–6–5–4–3–2–1.

I am perfectly and completely relaxed and comfortable, more relaxed than I have ever been before. All parts of my body are completely in tune with one another and totally relaxed and comfortable and pleasant. Everything about me is more relaxed and more comfortable than I have ever known before. This is a very pleasant sensation, nothing to worry about, perfectly safe.

I focus intensely upon my right hand. I repeat mentally: I feel only my right hand and no other part of my body. I allow my right hand to become lighter and lighter, and it feels as if my hand were being pulled up into the air, as if there were a big comfortable balloon lifting it up higher and higher into the air. My right hand is becoming lighter and lighter and lighter. My body is becoming more and more relaxed, breathing itself comfortably and relaxed and my right hand is rising higher and higher into the air. I don't have to strain. I allow it to happen by itself, feeling as if it were being pulled up by my body's relaxation, higher and higher, lighter and lighter, more and more comfortable. There is no rush to it.

It happens very slowly and very gently, very, very carefully. I allow my hand to become lighter and lighter, more and more comfortable, more and more pleasant as it does so. There is no strain in it, no hurry at all. My fingertips straighten out a little bit as they begin to lift up off the floor, off the chair. My right hand is becoming lighter and lighter, lifting higher and higher. I allow it to lift up on its own. I want it to happen. I don't have to do anything to allow it to happen. It will happen by itself. My right hand is lighter and lighter, more and more comfortable. All parts of my right hand are lighter and lighter and more and more relaxed and comfortable, rising up slowly and comfortably until it's straight up in the air over me. My right hand is lighter and lighter as if it were part of the air around me.

It is a very light and pleasant sensation to allow myself to relax like this. My right hand becomes easier and easier and higher and higher, lighter and lighter, more and more pleasant, rising up slowly and gently and gradually and pleasantly while all parts of my body are deeply relaxed and comfortable. My body breathes itself. My heartbeat is calm and regular; my right hand is becoming lighter and lighter as I allow it to rise up into the air as if it were being pulled up by a magnet. I don't resist it. I allow it to happen. It just wants to come up into the air by itself. It's getting lighter and lighter. My right hand is more and more comfortable, more and more a part of the air around me. My fingertips are lifting, straightening out, and becoming lighter and lighter, more and more comfortable.

All the parts of my body are relaxed, and my right hand is lifting up into the air as if it were joining a bird in flight, lighter and lighter, higher and higher. All the parts of my hand are now lifting up into the air, lighter and lighter, higher and higher. My body is more and more relaxed, and my right arm and hand are lighter and lighter, lifting up into the air more and more, very, very comfortable and relaxed. All parts of my body are relaxed and especially my right hand and arm are totally relaxed and comfortable and light, lifting up into the air, so comfortable that I feel as though there is no strain at all. It can hold itself there and doesn't need any muscle power to do it as my right hand lifts up into the air lighter and lighter, more and more comfortable, more relaxed and more comfortable than I have ever been at any time in my entire life.

All parts of my body are deeply and comfortably relaxed, especially my right hand and my right arm are totally relaxed, totally a part of the air about me lifting up and up and up, higher and higher above my body. My right hand is higher and higher, coming on up into the air higher and higher, more and more pleasant as my hand rises up. Each moment that I lift my hand and as it becomes higher and higher, my body becomes more and more relaxed, more and more comfortable, more relaxed than I have ever been at any time in my entire life. Higher and higher, and lighter and lighter. All the parts of my body are relaxed and comfortable, and my right hand and arm are especially relaxed and very, very light and comfortable, lifting up into the air, comfortable, relaxed and very, very light as if they were part of the air around me. Very, very light, very, very comfortable. All parts of my right hand lifting up, flying above my body, being drawn and pulled up, lighter and lighter, higher and higher into the air. All parts of my body are relaxed and comfortable.

When my hand has reached that stage, I allow it to become extremely light and then stiffen it out straight as a board. I tighten it up once again, very tight and stiff in the air. I straighten it out tightly, so stiff that it couldn't be bent. I straighten out that right arm as stiff as it can be. The rest of my body is perfectly relaxed, and my right arm is becoming stiffer and stiffer and stronger and stronger, all parts of my right arm totally stiff and strong and tight. [*Pause 15 seconds.*]

I relax now and allow my arm to fall back down beside me quickly and completely relaxed. My whole body is now more relaxed and more comfortable than it has ever been before. It has been a perfect exercise, a comfortable exercise which I have enjoyed doing. My body and mind working together like that, relaxed and in tune with one another. My entire body is perfectly, comfortably relaxed, totally in tune with itself. All parts of my body are totally relaxed and comfortable.

Now I feel my right hand again. I examine it and feel it mentally. I feel the blood pulsating gently through it, becoming warm, tingling, and I concentrate my attention entirely within my right hand. I feel my right hand intensely, strongly. I feel more from my right hand than I have ever felt before. I imagine that my entire mind and body are only in my right hand. I place all sensation within my right hand. I concentrate my attention there.

As I do so, my hand begins to expand in size. I allow it to become as big as I like. But as it does so, my hand will become numb, and I allow it to happen. I allow my hand to become number and number and less and less a part of my body. My right hand is becoming more and more numb, totally numb, totally without any feeling whatsoever. I am very aware of the place where my hand is, but I don't feel the hand itself. It's as if I felt only down to the wrist, my right hand becoming more and more numb. I am less and less aware of my right hand, and more and more aware of the absence of it. There is a loss of sensation of all kinds from my right hand; my right hand is becoming more and more numb, less and less a part of me, distracting my attention away from my hand to the point that I no longer feel it. It's no longer a part of my body. My right hand is totally separated from my mind and my body, becoming more and more numb, less and less a part of me. I feel only an absence of my right hand; it is free of movement, temperature, tingling; only numbness, as if it were totally absent.

I am feeling quite numb in my right hand and my entire body is becoming more and more relaxed, more and more comfortable. All parts of my body are more and more relaxed, more and more comfortable than I have ever been at any time in my life. My right hand is especially comfortable because it is totally numb. It's floating off in space distant from me. My body is still here totally relaxed and comfortable, but my right hand is totally absent, numb, free of all sensation.

Now I reach over with my left hand and feel for the place where my right hand was. I *feel* that my right hand is numb. As I touch my right hand with my left hand, it has much less feeling. My right hand is numb. My left hand feels normal. My right hand is totally free of sensation. I run my fingers over it. I can pinch it, and it's numb, very, very numb and very comfortable.

I put my left hand back down and allow my body to be more and more relaxed, more and more comfortable, more comfortable than it's ever been at any time before. I breathe deeply and comfortably, pleasantly. My heartbeat is calm and regular. All parts of my body are totally and equally relaxed, very comfortable and very relaxed.

Gradually, I allow the sensation to return to my right hand and as I do so, my right hand begins to tingle a little bit, and turn warmer. I feel my heart beating in it carrying sensation and warmth, oxygen and food to my right hand. My body is relaxed and all parts of my body are totally relaxed, totally comfortable, a very, very pleasant sensation. All parts of my body are very relaxed and very comfortable. All the parts are equally in tune with one another and with my mind. All parts of my body are beautifully and comfortably relaxed, more than they have ever been at any time in my entire life.

While I am in this state of mind now, I am capable of making mental trips. I allow my body to maintain itself in total comfort and relaxation, breathing itself, my heart beating calmly and regularly, and in my mind's eye, I visualize the most pleasant place I have ever known. I imagine that I am there. Suddenly, I transport myself in my mind's eye to my very favorite spot of relaxation and joy, wherever it may be—maybe on a mountain or at the seashore, in a forest, in a garden, wherever it may be, my favorite spot. I see myself relaxing and enjoying my favorite area. I can hear the sounds of that area and see the things that are going on there and smell all the things that I might find there, whether it's the sea or flowers. I may hear the birds chirping, I visualize it, I hear it, I feel myself traveling to this area safely and com-

fortably and pleasantly. I feel myself totally relaxed, totally within my perfect place of relaxation
and joy, and I abide there. I rest there, enjoy the
scenes that I see. I allow eight hours to pass.
[*Pause 2 minutes.*]

Now I picture myself, my entire body and mind,
functioning perfectly and normally, all parts of my
body and mind functioning comfortably and normally. I am relaxed.

Now I repeat over and over my own special healing affirmation. As I do so I see myself accomplishing my goal. [*Pause 5 minutes.*]

I am still in my favorite place of total joy and
relaxation, and have passed eight hours of total
pleasure there. It's time to come back into the
present, back into my totally comfortable and relaxed body. All the parts of my body are beautifully and comfortably in tune with my mind, totally comfortably relaxed and refreshed, just as if I
had had eight hours of sleep. I take another deep,
comfortable breath, and very, very slowly, I open
my eyes. [*Pause one minute.*] I look around
and I know that I am here, wide awake, refreshed,
comfortable and happy. I take a big pleasant
stretch, feeling the energy flowing throughout my
body.

AGE REGRESSION AND ATTUNEMENT

Relax. Close your eyes. Take a deep breath and
relax. Now repeat after me each phrase. [*Pause
15 seconds after each.*]

My arms and legs are heavy and warm. [*3 times*]

My heartbeat is calm and regular. [*3 times*]

My body breathes itself. [*3 times*]

My abdomen is warm. [*3 times*]

My forehead is cool. [*3 times*]

My mind is quiet and still. [*3 times*]

I am at peace.

Now I see and feel myself floating gently up into the air, out of this building, and up into the sky, 500 feet into the air. I am safe and happy and perfectly in control. I float in space and time, traveling wherever I wish. [*Pause 3 minutes.*]

Now I settle back into myself here. I relax and take a deep, pleasant, relaxing breath.

I will count backward now, seeing myself at the count of one projected to age 18. 20–19–18–17–16 . . . 1. I see myself now at my happiest experience at age 18. [*Pause 2 minutes.*] And I enjoy completely the great pleasures of being 18. I recapture the joy and optimism of age 18. I see the peace and freedom of that age. [*Pause 2 minutes.*]

I will count backward now, seeing myself at the count of one projected to age 12. 20–19–18–17–16 . . . 1. I see myself now at my pleasantest experience at age 12. [*Pause 2 minutes.*] And I enjoy completely the great pleasures of being age 12. I recapture the joy and optimism of age 12. I see the peace and freedom of that age. [*Pause 2 minutes.*]

I will count backward now, seeing myself at the count of one projected to age 6. 20–19–18–17–16 . . . 1. I see myself now at the most beautiful experience of age 6. [*Pause 2 minutes.*] And I enjoy completely the great pleasures of myself at age 6. I recapture the joy and optimism of age 6. I see the peace and freedom of that age. [*Pause 2 minutes.*]

I will count backward now, seeing myself at the count of one projected to age 3. 20–19–18–17–16– . . . 1. I see myself now at the happiest event of age 3. [*Pause 2 minutes.*] And I enjoy com-

pletely the great pleasures of myself at age 3. I
recapture the joy and optimism of age 3. I see the
peace and freedom of that age. [*Pause 2 minutes.*]

I will count backward now, seeing myself at the
count of one projected to my current age. 20–19–
18–17–16– . . . 1. I see myself now at my current
age and I completely enjoy the greatest pleasures
of being my current age. I recognize the loving,
happy nature of my inner self. I see and feel myself healthy and happy. [*Pause 2 minutes.*]

Now I repeat over and over my own special healing affirmation. As I do so I see myself accomplishing my goal. [*Pause 5 minutes.*]

Now as I prepare to return to my normal level of
awareness, I feel myself bringing with me the
health, happiness, and love I feel and see. I take a
deep, pleasant breath, open my eyes, and stretch
my entire body, feeling myself filled with loving
energy.

ROY MASTERS'S MEDITATION EXERCISE*

Sit comfortably with your hand hanging beside
you. Close your eyes. Take a deep comfortable
breath. Breathe deeply, slowly in and out. I am
going to teach you to concentrate. Listen very,
very carefully, repeat with me, follow the instructions and bring your attention to your hand beside
you.

Now repeat after me, silently, to yourself. I feel
the blood flowing down into my hand; it will
tingle. I just do that. I feel the blood flowing down
into my fingertips; I am conscious of my hand. I
am very, very conscious of my hand; I shift atten-

*I particularly appreciate Mr. Roy Masters's permission to print our
version of his exercise from his book *How Your Mind Can Keep
You Well* (Foundation Books, 1972). I have altered his technique
from second person ("you") to first person ("I") to emphasize *self*-
involvement.

tion from one finger to another. I do not lift my hand purposefully. I do not physically move my hand; I feel my hand. I focus my attention on my thumb, then my second finger, third, fourth, and fifth, and back to my thumb again. I am very, very aware of each finger in turn until I feel as though the blood were flowing down into it.

The object of this exercise is to cause my arm to become very, very light by concentrating fully on its lightness. While I am being very, very aware of my hand, at the same time—and I *can* do it—I make a mental picture of the back of my hand touching the middle of my forehead. I picture the back of my hand touching the middle of my forehead. If my mind wanders off, I bring my attention back to my hand. My awareness of my hand makes it tingle, as though the blood were flowing down into it.

Then again I form a mental picture of my hand going up toward the middle of my forehead. I keep doing it, I don't stop. I am very, very aware of my hand. I am very conscious of it. I feel the presence of my hand. I feel the blood flowing down into my hand, and then out of this feeling I find I can make a mental picture of my hand moving toward my head and my head moving toward my hand. If my thoughts wander off, I bring my attention back to my hand and then again feel the awareness, feel the presence of it and then make a mental picture of my hand, the back of my hand drawing up toward me, the back of my hand coming up to touch the middle of my forehead, as though I were looking out into space with my mind's eye. I am very conscious of the center of my forehead.

Then I feel the awareness of my hand and make a mental picture of my hand moving toward my head and of my head moving toward my hand. If my thoughts wander off, I feel the awareness of my hand again and then I make a mental picture of my hand drawing upward toward my head and of my head moving toward my hand. I keep doing it, I keep doing it, I don't stop. I think only of my hand rising up to touch my forehead. I judge the distance between my hand and the middle of my forehead. I estimate the distance. There is no hurry. I am patient. There is lots and lots of time. I am conscious of my hand. I feel my awareness of it. I make a mental picture of it coming toward me as if I were looking out through the middle of my forehead, drawing my hand closer and closer and closer, and I keep doing it. If my thoughts wander off, I bring my mind back to the awareness of my hand. I feel the blood flowing into my hand. I feel the presence of it and then I make a mental picture of my hand drawing toward the middle of my forehead as though I were looking out into space.

I can see it coming toward me, but I don't strain my eyes; I have the awareness, in the middle of my forehead, of my mind's eye. I don't squint with my eyes; I just observe as though I were looking out through the middle of my forehead, the place my thoughts arise, and I make a mental picture of the back of my hand drawing up toward me. I don't hurry.

The object of the exercise is to allow my arm to respond to my inner self, light and buoyant, as though my hand wished to move by itself. I allow my hand to rise. I know I can put my hand down any time I like. I just keep feeling as if my hand were rising up to touch my forehead. I just let my hand go up by itself; it may even feel as if I were fooling myself. If my mind wanders off, I bring my attention back to my hand, feel the awareness of my hand. I feel the tingling sensation as if the blood were flowing down into my fingers. I make a mental image of my hand coming toward the middle of my forehead as though I were looking out into space.

I do not strain. I am just very, very aware of the center of my forehead, and very, very aware of my hand rising up to touch my forehead. I find that I can dissolve unnecessary, unwanted thoughts in this fashion by becoming aware of the presence of my hand, just by being very aware of my hand rising up to touch my forehead. I feel it coming up toward my forehead. I feel it coming up toward me so that the back of my hand will touch the middle of my forehead. I can judge the distance. In my imagination, in my estimation, I can judge the distance between the back of my hand and the middle of my forehead. I draw my hand closer and closer.

I allow my hand to rise up and I feel in a few minutes that the back of my hand is closer to my forehead than it really is. I may think that if I move my hand just a little bit closer, the back of my hand will touch the middle of my forehead, but it hasn't yet. It feels as though my hand is passing through my head rather than to my head. I will just be aware of my hand rising higher and higher toward my forehead. At all times, I am aware of my hand. And when it does move a little closer, it doesn't really seem to get there. It seems as though it were closer than it really is. This is just an effect created by my own concentration.

Now I will just keep being aware of my hand. I will be very, very conscious of my hand. I feel the blood flowing into my hand; it will tingle. It may feel a little numb or detached, but I will just keep being aware of my hand and making a mental image of my hand coming toward me, coming closer and closer and closer until the back of my hand touches the middle of my forehead. I keep doing it. I keep doing it. I don't stop. I keep thinking of my hand. I am aware of my hand. I draw it closer to my forehead. When the back of my hand touches the middle of my forehead, I will leave it there until it becomes tired and then drop it beside me again.

And when I have done it with one hand, I will become aware of the other hand and do it with the other hand. Just for a few moments, I will keep concentrating on the place in the middle of my forehead, not with my eyes, but with my inner awareness. When my hand touches the middle of my forehead, I leave it there and leave it there as long as I can, but drop it when it is tired; then I continue to concentrate on the awareness of my hands as I seem to focus my attention on the middle of my forehead. I am very, very aware of the back of my hand touching the middle of my forehead. If it is not yet touching in the middle of my forehead, I will just keep being aware of my hand, very conscious of it. I keep feeling that tingling sensation, feeling as though the blood were flowing into it, and I keep on drawing my hand up toward the middle of my forehead.

Each time I do this exercise, I will be increasing my ability to observe, to control my thoughts from within myself, because the exercise makes it so. Each time I do this exercise, I keep being aware of my hand, I am creating a greater awareness of the present; the unpleasant events of the past become less and less important, dissolved in the light of reality, because the exercise makes it so. And I am very, very aware of my hand rising up to touch my forehead. I cannot change my past anyway so there is no point in thinking about it or being annoyed by it, no matter what it was. No longer does it feel, nor is it, important. There is nothing I can do in my thinking to change it, so I will forget it, and be very, very aware of my hand, rising up to touch the middle of my forehead. What I do not think about cannot bother me.

The future is similar. I will not worry about it. This exercise of being aware of my hand will cause me to keep my awareness in the present, because the exercise makes it so. The exercise will allow me to lose all thoughts except the awareness of my hand. It will clear my mind and cause me to keep in my thinking simple things that will be revealed to me in the place in my mind where I used to be annoyed but am no longer. And I will be very, very aware of my hand rising up to touch the center of my forehead. At all times, I am very, very aware of my hand rising up to touch the center of my forehead. Nothing from now on must upset, irritate, aggravate, agitate, or harm my feelings, not in the slightest degree, especially those little unkind, unfair, and dishonest things that people say and do to me and others from day to day. And I am very, very aware of my hand rising up to touch the center of my forehead. I will not be annoyed inwardly or outwardly. I will not suppress anger; I will just overlook and forgive problems that cannot be changed, make allowances immediately right at the moment, not because I have to but because I want to; and I am very, very aware of my hand rising up to touch the center of my forehead. At all times, I am aware of the presence of my hand rising up to touch the center of my forehead.

I realize it is my own anger and irritation that hurt me more than the unthinking cruelties of other people. Therefore, from now on, I will overlook, watch for the opportunity to overlook, and forgive right on the spot, not two seconds later but immediately when it happens so that I will respond more to what I know and shall come to know as right and less and less to conditions and people. And I am very, very aware of my hand rising up to touch the center of my forehead. I will make allowances for and forgive everyone from now on, no matter who it is, especially those close to me.

Since I cannot control my faults, those I can see and those I cannot, I do not have the right to be annoyed at the faults of others, especially my family. The ones to make allowances for first are the ones close to me. If I cannot do it for my

loved ones, how can I expect to do it for strangers
or how can I expect others to forgive me? If I
make allowances for my family, it will be easier
for me to do it for people who mean less to me. I
am very, very aware of my hand rising up to touch
the center of my forehead.

Love does not expect anything from anyone. It is
what I expect others to do and do not receive that
makes me annoyed. It does not matter what others
have or do. When I do something for someone, I
will do it because I want to, not because I have
to; and I am very, very aware of my hand rising
up to touch the center of my forehead.

I will have no imaginary conversations with people as to what I am going to say to so and so the
next time I see him or her. Never mind what I
should have done or could have done or said;
what has been cannot be changed, no matter how
much I wish it. But I can change from now on. I
am very, very aware of my hand rising up to
touch the center of my forehead.

If I have felt disturbed about some worry or mis-
take in the past, I will remember that those persons, if they are good, would have forgiven me
without my asking. If they are not good, I will
just start making allowances for and forgiving
them from now on; for it is written, "Forgive us
as we forgive others." That implies that each
time I am patient with another, I obtain forgive-
ness and salvation and I undo a few of my past
mistakes also. And I am very, very aware of my
hand rising up to touch the center of my forehead.

The coward is a coward from the time he should
have been brave until the next time. If he again
fails to be brave, he is a greater coward, and with
more remorse, than before, but if he chooses to be
brave and courageous at that time, he will no
longer be a coward. If the world should suddenly

become perfect, the coward would never have a chance to redeem himself. I am very, very aware of the presence of my hand rising up to touch the center of my forehead.

And so it is with me. I have allowed myself to become annoyed and irritated over many trivial things in life, and when I should have overlooked them or made allowances, I did not. I am very, very aware of my hand rising up to touch the center of my forehead.

If there were no danger, I could not possess courage. If there were no hatred nor temptation, how could I develop love and virtue? Other people are giving me an opportunity to accomplish now what I may have failed to do before. Situations which once made me upset, guilty and afraid, will become the very things to give me happiness and a sense of well-being from now on; and I am very, very aware of the presence of my hand rising up to touch the center of my forehead. Whosoever should try to anger me or upset me is giving me an opportunity to rise above my problems. They do not know this, but they are doing me a great favor and the harder people try to upset me, the calmer I will become; the brighter my light will shine. So I will remember, overlook, and forgive right on the spot, be plain spoken, tell the truth with firmness, kindness and patience from now on; and I am very, very aware of my hand rising up to touch the center of my forehead.

He who tends to annoy me, intentionally or otherwise, is trying to hurt and control me with my own anger. I will keep him out of my thoughts. I will respond only with patience and whatever thought or deed that shall come forth out of my center of calmness. I am very, very aware of my hand.

I keep this idea running through my thoughts often. I will have the awareness of it at all times in my mind. I will keep this as a spiritual and moral goal. I will let it be more important than any material goal in the world, for it is the means by which everything else can be accomplished. I will let the whole procedure give me a satisfaction and a joy of doing which will far exceed the pleasure from material things. It will be a joy to think about, to understand, and to do again and again. It will change everything that passes through my mind; and I am very, very aware of my hand rising up to touch the center of my forehead.

I shall make decisions according to my inner calmness. Everything I feel, do, or say will conform to it. That is, I will be patient, overlook and forgive, be outspoken with fairness, kindness, and patience; and I am very, very aware of my hand rising up to touch the center of my forehead.

I do it because I want to, not because I have to. I do it because I want understanding. I do it for the sake of honesty rather than to feel good. I do it for the pure love of seeing truth prevail, to be a better person regardless of profit or loss or whether it makes me well, and I am very, very aware of my hand rising up to touch the center of my forehead.

If I want to have a real goal to think about, I will let it be just to learn to be unmoving in my patience and to make allowances for others. If I could do that, I would truly be better off. The achievement of no other goal could give me such satisfaction. Everything I am saying merely points to the simplest instruction to overlook and forgive on the spot and to be plainspoken with firmness, kindness, and patience; and I am very, very aware of my hand rising up to touch the center of my forehead.

Part of this conversation is helping me understand; the other is directing me to think, feel, and act so that I know how to use my calm inner peace. This is very important. I will remember it often. I will do this exercise on my own and I will find it keeps the thought alive; and I am very, very aware of my hand rising up to touch my forehead.

If I have something to say, I will say it. If I have something to do, I will do it. What isn't worth saying or doing isn't worth thinking about, so I will forget it. As long as I am calm and patient and not upset, I cannot possibly hurt anyone with my words or deeds and at those times I have a right to speak up. I cannot please everyone anyway, so I will stop trying that. I am responsible only for expressing the truth for each moment. If others become upset over my purity, then they will see their own faults in the light of my patience; and I am very, very aware of my hand rising up to touch the center of my forehead.

The first thing is to react only after careful thought, never jumping to conclusions. I will be patient under trial. As long as I am not annoyed, I will always be able to disagree without being disagreeable. If people are upset because of my honesty, they are not my friends anyway; and I might as well know it. My real friends will come to respect me and love me for my honesty and truthfulness; and I am very, very aware of my hand rising up to touch the center of my forehead.

I will not plan my conversations ahead of time, such as "If he says this to me, I will say that to him." I will keep the idea pure in my mind. Whatever it is, I will overlook pettinesses and forgive. I will be plainspoken with firmness, kindness, and patience. I will make sure that I overlook the things that should be overlooked, and that I am plainspoken about those things that should be said. I will use my judgment; and I am very, very aware of the presence of my hand, the tingle of blood flowing through my hand. At all times I feel my hand rising up to touch the center of my forehead.

I will be sure not to change my words just to soften the outcome, keeping within myself that which should be said or done and which may fester into resentment or guilt if not expressed. Whatever personal problem I have, I will stop looking for a reason, for I will see the reason in good time. All I achieve by searching is to confuse myself even more. I will keep problems out of my thoughts by dwelling on what I am learning at this moment; and I am very, very aware of my hand rising up to touch the center of my forehead.

I will not analyze what I am thinking; I will only push additional thoughts out of my mind. I will just be aware of my hand rising up to touch the center of my forehead. I will just keep relating to and remembering the basic premise, which is to rise above pettiness and forgive on the spot and to be plainspoken and honest. It does not matter whether others love me, if I love them. It does not matter if people understand me, if I understand them. And, if they do not forgive me, I forgive them. And I am very, very aware of my hand rising up to touch the center of my forehead.

I will not say "Stupid idiot!" when someone else acts foolishly; rather I will say, to myself, "Here, let me help you." Although it is correct to observe faults, I will not puff up emotionally and criticize others. I will make allowances and forgive them on the spot. I will not take personal offense at anything. I will let criticism roll off me like water off a duck's back. I will not be excited by praise or offended by criticism; and I am very, very aware of my hand rising up to touch the center of my forehead.

I will do it because I want to, not because I have to. I will remember to understand and forgive on the spot and to be outspoken with firmness, kindness, and patience, keeping the theme uppermost in my thoughts. I will not worry about nor dwell upon the past or the future; and I am very, very aware of my hand rising up to touch the center of my forehead.

I will do this exercise by myself, and this exercise will furnish the energy to keep this understanding alive, which is to be patient and plainspoken, and at all times to be very, very aware of my hand rising up to touch the center of my forehead.

Each time I am patient and do not respond to torment and temptation, there will be a great feeling of achievement and I will see things in a different light, and what I shall come to understand will increase the meaning of the basic truth which is to understand and forgive on the spot.

Then, each time I do my exercise, I will automatically carry down my new understanding into my daily life so that I will do it with increasing skill, which in turn will bring more understanding; and the more I understand, the more I will feel inclined to do what I do understand, and the less I will respond to outer conditions, to temptation, and to what other people say and do. I will respond only to my inner self and be very, very aware of my hand rising up to touch the center of my forehead.

Nothing will be added to this idea while I am doing the exercise, nor anything taken away from it. I will merely be reminded to understand and forgive on the spot, to be outspoken with firmness, kindness, and patience and be very aware of my hand, rising up to touch the center of my forehead.

I did not say that I cannot think of anything else. As I go through my daily chores and come into contact with people, no matter what I do, no matter what I feel and think, I will do everything in accordance with the instructions to understand and forgive on the spot, to be outspoken with firmness, kindness, and patience from now on; and be very, very aware of my hand rising up to touch the center of my forehead.

I will remember to make allowances for people with all my thinking, all my feeling, with all my understanding, with all my being, because I want to, not because I have to. And I am very, very aware of the presence of my hand rising up to touch the center of my forehead.

I will not analyze, ponder on it within myself; I will not worry, will it work, will it last? I will cast out all doubt. I will bring my mind back again and again to my objective. I will not discuss this, or even think about it; I will just feel it within and do it and be very, very aware of the presence of my hand rising up to touch the center of my forehead. I continue to relax and be very, very aware of my hand. I relax and allow my body to breathe comfortably.

Now slowly, as I complete this exercise, I allow my hand to fall gently beside me. And I recognize that I am helping my body heal itself by having it respond in this way, by having my body and mind work together in perfect harmony. And as I return to a normal level of awareness, I bring back with me the beautiful sensation of comfort, relaxation, and joy felt at the deeper levels of thinking I have experienced. I take a deep breath, open my eyes, and stretch comfortably, feeling the energy flowing throughout my body.

WISE MAN ATTUNEMENT

Before we begin, spend 2 minutes thinking of the three most important questions in your life—specific questions about yourself, questions that can be answered in a few sentences, such as "What is my most important goal?" or "How can I best use my spare time?" *Pause 2 minutes.*

Relax. Close your eyes. Take a deep breath and relax. Now repeat after me each phrase. [*Pause 15 seconds after each.*]

My arms and legs are heavy and warm. [*3 times*]

My heartbeat is calm and regular. [*3 times*]

My body breathes itself. [*3 times*]

My abdomen is warm. [*3 times*]

My forehead is cool. [*3 times*]

My mind is quiet and still. [*3 times*]

I am at peace.

Now I visualize myself climbing up a beautiful mountain at night. I see a full moon and a clear path winding upward. I smell the woods. I hear crickets chirping and birds singing. I am coming closer and closer to the top of the mountain. As I walk up, I enter a clearing and see a pleasant fire burning. Sitting behind the fire is a wise man, who appears very kind and peaceful. I approach and place another log on the fire. As I sit down I introduce myself to the wise man. We sit and chat together for a while. [*Pause 3 minutes.*]

Now I ask the wise man my third most important question. [*Pause 3 minutes.*]

I ask the wise man my second most important question, and I listen carefully to his answer. [*Pause one minute.*]

I ask the wise man my most important question, and I listen and understand his answer. [*Pause 3 minutes.*]

As I prepare to say good night, the wise man reaches into a leather sack and gives me a special personal gift. I examine it carefully in the moonlight. I embrace the wise man lovingly as we part. As I walk back down the path, I feel happy, joyful, loving, and healthy. And I know I can visit with the wise man again, at any time I like. The wise man can always help to answer my questions.

Now I repeat over and over my own special healing affirmation. As I do so I see myself accomplishing my goal. [*Pause 5 minutes.*]

As I prepare to return to my normal level of awareness, I feel myself bringing with me the health and the happiness and love that I feel and see. I take a deep breath, open my eyes, stretch comfortably, and feel myself filled with loving energy.

CREATING YOUR OWN PROGRAM TO HEAL YOURSELF

Considering the unique individuality of each person, there is no way I can cover every possible problem, but you know your own needs and can adapt the general principles covered in this book to assist you in your personal program. One of the first requirements is development of your own special phrase. In the exercises, I have referred often to "your own special healing phrase." Your phrase might be directed toward correction of physical, emotional or spiritual deficits. It may be general, such as "Every day in every way I am getting better and better," "becoming more and more healthy," "more and more wealthy." Or it may be quite specific such as some of the "organ specific" phrases to be suggested later.

Now is the ideal time to assess your strengths and weaknesses. Sit down, relax, separate yourself from your emotions and write out a list which includes at least these items. Reassess your list once every month for three months, then two or three times a year.

	My Major: Weaknesses	Strengths	Goals
Physical:	1. 2. 3. 4.		
Emotional:	1. 2. 3. 4.		
Financial:	1. 2. 3. 4.		
Work:	1. 2. 3. 4.		
Family:	1. 2. 3. 4.		
Spiritual:	1. 2. 3. 4.		

Now review these carefully to make a conscious decision concerning those you wish to enhance or improve. Then write phrases for accomplishing your goals. And with each phrase, create an *image*—imagine yourself achieving your goal. Work on one or two at a time or try creating a composite, short, positive phrase and image which includes all the desired goals. Picture yourself as you will be when you have reached your goals. Make this *your* special healing phrase. In addition to using it during the three Biogenics practice sessions each day, incorporate your phrase in other daily activities. For instance, chant it to yourself while you do your physical limbering or strengthening exercises.

Establish a habit of reaffirming your phrase at least once each hour by closing your eyes (in a safe spot, of course), breathing deeply and slowly 10 times while you repeat your phrase. This 2½-minute "break" will help refresh and remotivate you and allow you to work at a more consistent productive pace. Remember, "Every thought is a prayer," as Ambrose Worrall so beautifully discussed in *Essay on Prayer*. To what are you praying? Direct your thoughts—prayers—toward your ideals!

Focus your attention upon your capacity for compassion, wisdom, understanding, and love. Create your own reality.

The following are generalized phrases which may be of help in deciding upon your healing phrase.

1) I live every moment of every day with full vitality and love.

2) I feel myself close to the earth, flowers, trees, grass, clouds, rain, wind, sky, sun and stars.

3) I feel a sense of deep inner energy, strength, power, well-being, self-confidence, and peace.

4) I feel myself bathed in the golden light of Universal Love.

5) Life is beautiful, for God's spirit is within me.

6) I am calmer each day.

7) I am younger each day.

8) I am wealthier each day.

9) I am more motivated each day.

10) Every day I have greater faith in myself and in God.

As a final consideration, if you already have or do develop specific illnesses, develop your own special program along the general outlines which have been presented. These may be organ specific or disease specific. In general, one would use deep relaxation, followed by repetition of the appropriate phrase, always a proper positive statement concerning the desired physiological and physical change, and appropriate *visualization* of the body and the particular area as being healthy. Be certain always to use only positive statements. Never say "don't." Here are some examples:

For rheumatoid arthritis:

My joints are flexible and comfortable.

My joints are normally cool and relaxed.

For high blood pressure:

My blood pressure is 120/80.

My blood pressure is perfectly normal.

For asthma:

My breathing is always free, relaxed, and comfortable.

For multiple sclerosis:

My immune system is perfectly balanced.

My nerve tissue is joyously healthy.

For hardening of the arteries:

My arteries are soft and normally open.

My cholesterol is perfectly normal.

My circulation is perfectly balanced.

For epilepsy:

My brain is perfectly coordinated.

The electrical activity of my brain is always calm and relaxed.

For any blood chemistry abnormality:

My [*name the blood chemistry*] is perfectly normal.

For hormonal problems:

>My glandular functions are perfectly balanced.
>
>My [*name the gland*] functions perfectly.

For colds, flu, and sore throat:

>My immune system protects me from all infections.
>
>My nose and throat are warm and healthy.
>
>I am comfortably filled with perfect, loving energy.

For anxiety, undue fear:

>I am relaxed and comfortable.
>
>I am calm and serene.
>
>I am safe and happy.

For obesity:

>My appetite is pleasantly satisfied.
>
>I am desirably thin.

For cancer healing:

Use any 5-to-10 minute induction of relaxation, physiological balance, mental balancing, spiritual attunement. Then repeat:

>I visualize my immune system as strong and healthy. [*10 times*]
>
>My immune system protects me perfectly from all cancer cells. [*10 times*]
>
>My body is continuously healing itself. [*10 times*]
>
>I see myself filled and surrounded by universal light and love. [*10 times*]
>
>And I bring back with me this feeling and vision of love.

I take a deep breath, open my eyes, breathe out, and stretch comfortably feeling myself filled with loving energy.

And, of course, once again, if you are ill or become ill, your own physician is still your best bet for diagnosis and recommendations.

ELEVEN

Pain

One of the most important messages of Biogenics is that you must learn to *listen to,* to *feel,* each part of your body, and then to create—through words, images, and self-love—the proper balance in each organ or area as well as the integration of the whole. Biogenics helps, through insight and relaxation, to balance dependent-passive needs with freedom-aggressive ones, to integrate love for self with love for humanity. You need to listen to and recognize negative emotions so that you can take conscious, positive action to resolve conflicts. The goal is the harmonization of will and imagination, the conscious mind with the subconscious.

Anxiety, depression, fear, anger, and guilt are messages from the subconscious that all is not well. Pain is a similar message from the body, but one that generally implies physical damage or the threat of damage. If we listen to the message carefully, we may learn either that disease or injury exists, or that we are ignoring that part of the body, failing to integrate it into our total body-mind image, or that we are reacting symbolically to frustration or suppressed emotions, such as when we find ourselves saying, "He's a pain in the neck," or "She's on my back."

Despite the preponderance of pain as the most

common symptom presented to physicians, in and of itself it still receives remarkable little general medical attention as anything but a symptom of a disease that must be diagnosed and is not ordinarily given any specific place in medical school curricula. It is not surprising then that most physicians are more frustrated by their attempts to manage pain than by any other patient problem. During the last decade, considerable progress in pain management has been achieved and has even led to the development of a new medical specialty: dolorology. Currently, there are three full-time dolorologists plus a number of physicians who spend 30 percent or more of their time in dolorology. It is hoped that many more physicians will come to consider pain management a worthwhile career.

Since most sicknesses involve pain, let's take a closer look at it as a disturbance of health.

CAUSES OF PAIN

Physical. Excessive pressure upon or damage to almost any body tissue leads to pain. Trauma, scar, hemorrhage, infection, herniated tissue, and tumors are all causes of such physical alterations.

Physiological. This category includes pain caused by muscle spasm, exposure to extremes of heat (42° C. or above) or cold (less than 10° C.), inflammation, and autonomic dysfunction. In fact, most pain includes, as an initiating factor or as a reaction to injury, a disturbance of the autonomic nervous system. Such alterations lead to vascular and/or biochemical disturbances that may induce pain.

Disturbances perpetuating chronic pain even though the initial cause may be removed include:

(1) Various types of nerve damage (degenerative, traumatic, infectious, vascular, or chemical): often patients who have lost an arm or leg (phantom limb) or even had total destruction of a portion of the spinal cord (paraplegia) hurt in the "numb" or absent areas. Such pain arises from an imbalance in the normal sensory nerves. Normally the larger nerve fibers, beta, carry non-painful information such as touch or

vibration; but their major function seems to be to regulate or balance the total input to the spinal cord and ultimately to the brain. Loss of beta fibers may, then, allow messages from the smallest, C, fibers to get through unimpeded and create feelings of pain. Patients who hurt for months or years after shingles, for example, have a greater loss of beta fibers than of C fibers.

(2) Anatomical disordering of the autonomic nervous system by injury or surgery.

Psychological. Anxiety and most other emotional distress upset the autonomic nervous system setting the stage for a tremendous variety of psychosomatic or psychophysiological disturbances capable in themselves of inducing pain and perpetuating it. Peptic ulcer and asthma fit into this category—not to mention all those diseases not yet commonly recognized as being caused by stress.

THERAPY FOR PAIN

Clearly, the first step you take whenever you develop pain or any other symptom of illness, is to consult your physician for the proper diagnosis. Then you and he or she together will work to overcome the distress. For your general knowledge, here are some common methods used to treat pain. It's only with a doctor's advice, of course, that any of these should be used.

Acupuncture. Whatever its mechanism of action, acupuncture is physiologically helpful in relieving both acute and chronic pain.

Narcotics. In acute pain of most sorts, narcotics offer effective and rapid pain relief, but not without such potential undesirable effects as nausea, mental confusion, hypotension, respiratory depression, and—addiction. In chronic pain they are not effective and are not indicated.

Synthetic Analgesics. Despite many introductions in the past two decades (Darvon®, Empirin®, Ponstel®, Talwin®, and so on) no non-narcotic has been proved more effective than aspirin. Injectable Talwin® is a dangerous and highly addictive drug and should be abandoned. Even Tylenol® is probably more useful than Darvon. But all such drugs are quite limited in their usefulness in chronic pain.

Tranquilizers. Despite their widespread use (they are prescribed more than any other drugs), there is no evidence that any tranquilizer is of significant benefit in managing pain. Furthermore, they alter personality and brain function and are specifically *not* indicated.

Antidepressants. In addition to successfully treating depression, the so-called tricyclic compounds, especially Elavil®, have been effective in relieving some pain problems caused by nerve damage. Occasionally Dilantin® may also help. However, such side effects as rashes, low blood pressure, mental confusion or euphoria, or urinary and bladder difficulties prevent the use of Elavil® in about 25 percent of patients.

Heat. Local heat has long been used for relieving pain. It is particulary useful for pain accompanying muscular spasm.

Ice. Rubdowns with ice or use of commercial ice packs, such as Therapac®, are useful in reducing pain. Acute pain responds much more commonly than does chronic pain, but overall, ice is even better than heat.

Massage. Both focal and generalized massages are often useful in reducing muscular spasm and also in achieving greater flexibility and relaxation.

External Electrical Stimulation. Battery-powered, pulsed electric current applied on either side of a painful area or over a major nerve trunk serving the area of pain is known to relieve pain in most acute situations (80 percent) and in some chronic ones (25 percent). It is probably the best simple mechanical treatment of all those mentioned. However, special technicians or trained nurses are needed for effective use of this approach. It is particularly valuable in postoperative management where temporary paralysis of the intestines or partial collapse of lungs from poor breathing can be practically abolished. Someday I hope every home has such a device available for application after fresh injuries. The total amount of pain can be reduced and recovery speeded up by external electrical stimulation.

Autogenic Training and Biofeedback. For acute pain, hypnosis is an excellent therapeutic approach, but it is generally successful in only 25 percent of the patients for whom it is attempted. In cases of chronic pain, it is not often of lasting benefit. Although more time consuming than any other technique mentioned, Biogenics—verbal self-regulatory training—offers the most effective therapy for all chronic pain states. Eighty percent of those patients who will practice for six months or longer gain marked to total pain relief. The initial training requires 12 hours for migraine to 60 hours for other pains.

Nerve Blocks. In addition to their familiar use as local anesthetics, various types of nerve blocks, such as Novocaine®, are useful as diagnostic aids and occasionally are adequate therapy in acute pain; rarely, however, will repeated blocks alleviate chronic pain.

Destructive Neurosurgical Procedures. With few exceptions, destruction of peripheral nerves or parts of the spinal cord or brain have been of little value in the management of pain. Cutting the fifth cranial nerve is most useful for tic douloureux (painful facial neuralgia); and occasionally nerves are cut for chest pain that is due to a fractured vertebra. Cordotomy, cutting of the spinal cord, should be done only for unilateral cancer pain. Destruction of spinal facet joint nerves has been quite useful in many patients with back and sciatic pain and is quite safe. Various destructive procedures in the brain (lobotomy, cingulumotomy, thalamotomy, for instance) are of no value in benign pain but may on rare occasion be recommended for cancer pain.

Physical Exercise. After the first month or so of healing of an injury or a surgical wound, progressive physical limbering and strengthening are essential for comfort. Prolonged inactivity is usually harmful and should be vigorously opposed.

MANAGEMENT OF PAIN

1. Obtain a proper diagnosis.

2. Correct physical disturbances whenever possible. However, once surgery has failed, repeated surgery is rarely indicated.

3. In acute pain, consider—
   a. Ice
   b. External electrical stimulation
   c. Narcotics (but used only on a time-regulated basis. Never use "on demand" or "as needed" for longer than a week; do not use at all for longer than a month.)
   d. Acupuncture
   e. Nerve-block drugs such as Novocaine®
   f. Aspirin

4. In chronic pain, use—
   a. External electrical stimulation
   b. Ice
   c. Acupuncture
   d. Physical limbering and strengthening
   e. Biogenics
   f. Aspirin

Except in the most unusual circumstances, always avoid narcotics, tranquilizers, and multiple surgery. And *remember, at least 85 percent of the factors responsible for health are self-regulated and under your potential management.*

PAIN RELIEF THROUGH BIOGENICS

As you practice autogenic training you gradually learn that you have entered an altered state of feeling and awareness, in which *no* body sensations are felt and in which your mind is fantastically alert. You are perfectly, ideally conscious, and your mind seems capable of answering any question. If your EEG were being taken at such a time you would be in a slow, steady brain rhythm (alpha or theta). Repeated verbal and visual programming in this state of body–mind harmony will produce greater and greater freedom from pain. Such comfort will then be carried over into your normal states of activity for longer and longer periods of time, until you achieve consistent pain relief. Repeated practice is essential and may require 6 to 10 months of practicing 4 to 12 hours a day when the pain is severe.

The following exercise is excellent for inducing the state of deep relaxation and total body numbness or absence of all sensation in which programming for freedom from pain can be most effective.

Now relax, close your eyes, take a deep breath, and repeat mentally to yourself each sentence, feeling the sensation as you say:

My arms and legs are heavy and warm. [*6 times*]

My heartbeat is calm and regular. [*6 times*]

My body breathes itself freely and comfortably. [*6 times*]

My abdomen is warm. [*6 times*]

My forehead is cool. [*6 times*]

My mind is quiet and still. [*3 times*]

My mind is quiet and happy. [*3 times*]

I am at peace.

I feel my feet expanding lightly and pleasantly by one inch. [*2 times*]

My feet are now expanding lightly and pleasantly by 12 inches. [*2 times*]

The pleasant 12-inch expansion is spreading throughout all the parts of my legs. [*2 times*]

My abdomen, buttocks, and back are expanding 12 inches lightly and pleasantly. [*2 times*]

My chest is expanding 12 inches pleasantly and lightly. [*2 times*]

My arms and hands are expanding 12 inches lightly and pleasantly. [*2 times*]

My neck and head are joining in the 12 inches of expansion. [*2 times*]

My entire body is relaxed, expanded, and comfortable. [*6 times*]

My mind is quiet and still. [*2 times*]

I withdraw my mind from my physical surroundings. [*2 times*]

I am free of all physical sensations. [*2 times*]

I am free of all sensations. [*6 times*]

My body is safe and comfortable. [*3 times*]

My mind is quiet and still. [*3 times*]

Each time I practice this exercise my body becomes more and more comfortable. And I carry this comfort with me to my normal awareness.

I am relaxed and comfortable. [*3 times*]

I see and feel myself filled with universal love. [*3 times*]

And I will carry this love with me throughout each day.

I am attuned to my highest spiritual self. [*3 times*]

Each time I practice these exercises, I benefit more and more.

Every day in every way I am becoming healthier and healthier.

Now I repeat over and over my own personal healing affirmation. As I do so I see myself accomplishing my goal. [*Pause 5 minutes.*]

I am relaxed and comfortable. [*4 times*] [*Wait one minute.*]

I bring the comfort and relaxation achieved at this level of mental activity with me as I return to my normal level of awareness.

As I open my eyes, I take another deep relaxing breath and a big comfortable stretch, and feel myself filled with perfect, loving energy.

TWELVE

Health Versus Disease

True health is a state of balance of one's spiritual, mental, and physical elements, no one of which can be ignored without loss of balance.

Spiritual implies the realization of and attunement with one's ideal higher self and with the power of the universe, of God, if you will. Mental balance requires the dispassionate release of the negative feelings of fear, anger, guilt, hatred, hostility, frustration, and depression, which, when dispersed, will leave room for the love that will bring happiness, joy, and contentment:* Both spiritual and mental harmony are enhanced by such esthetic experiences as music, religion, appreciation of nature, and art.

Balance must include proper nutrition, relaxation, physical exercise—both limbering and strengthening—sanitation, immunization and treatment of illness, and exposure to light.

At the present time, most countries in our so-called civilized world, in fact, do not have a system of maintenance of good health; instead, they focus on the treatment of diseases. In the United States, we

---

*But you must consciously cultivate this love!

187

have an excellent system of sanitation and immunization and infectious diseases have been largely brought under control, but there is no other significant practice of preventive medicine or general health maintenance. Since Hippocrates, physicians have traditionally worked with the sick; rarely have they devoted much effort to working with the well to maintain their good health. The Chinese and many primitive tribes seem to have done a much better job of practicing health maintenance than Western society. Eastern philosophy, while emphasizing spiritual development and mental peace, has largely ignored the importance of physical health. Indeed, the Eastern diet is often as incomplete, with the lack of proper balanced protein, as is the Western, with its overprocessed foods and emphasis on sugar content.

Unfortunately, what passes in the United States as a system for health care is a disease-treatment system backed by "insurance," most of which covers the costs of only hospitalization and the illnesses that require it—and in many cases not a large percentage of those. (Although 9 out of 10 people under sixty-five have health insurance, only 4 out of 10 have major medical policies and only one person in 30 has dental insurance.) Such regulations, of course, have been largely responsible for the increased use of hospitals for ailments that can really be treated in the doctor's office.

If, however, intensive medical treatment is indicated, here are some pointers to remember.

HOSPITALIZATION

Avoid it if possible. I estimate that over 50 percent of hospitalized Americans are there primarily to claim the insurance payments. This is ridiculous. You're endangering your health and life and tripling and quadrupling the cost of medical care for everyone. Overdiagnosis, overtreatment, overmedication are "killing American medicine," according to Dr. Lawrence L. Weed, professor of medicine at the University of Vermont.* And the more hospital beds there are the more they are used! Even a conservative estimate reports that "25 percent of the patient population is treated in facilities excessive of their needs."†

Do try to go to the best hospital possible in cases of acute or emergency illness and very grave and serious ailments and injuries.

SURGERY

At least 50 percent of all surgery done in the United States is neither necessary nor indicated. In an emergency situation, you have little time to fool around, but with all elective surgery, including diagnostic surgery, ask yourself—

1. Is it necessary?

2. What are the risks—all of them and with what frequency?

3. What are the risks without surgery?

4. What are the alternatives to surgery?

Finally, get second and third opinions. It will pay you to have three independent surgeons advise you in relation to any elective surgery. Incidentally, this is especially essential with regard to a back operation. Back pain, with or without sciatica, often responds to such treatment as acupuncture, applications of ice, massage, manipulation, and external electrical stimulation, which should always be tried before surgery is considered. The exception is where there is significant weakness of the ability to raise the foot associated with the pain, which indicates nerve pressure.

If surgery is indicated, have it done under local anesthesia (but not a spinal) if at all possible. The rate of complications is lessened and your chances for sat-

---

Medical Group News 7 (July 1974):1, 4.
†"Let's Get Rid of Those Surplus Hospital Beds," *Prism* 2 (Oct. 1974): 13–14, 58, 60–61.

isfactory recovery are improved. Practice Biogenics intensely before, during, and after the surgery. Visualize yourself as recovering perfectly, rapidly.

DRUGS

Avoid them if possible. Complications, patronizingly called "side effects" by drug companies, can be fatal. Most drugs have a wide variety of complications, including nausea, dizziness, mental confusion, rashes, liver damage, and anemia (bone-marrow depression). Always ask:

1. *What are the risks? And get percentages.*

2. *What are the risks if I don't take this drug?*

3. *Is there any alternative?*

4. *Are there any interrelations with other drugs I'm taking? (It's best to ask a pharmacist or two this last question!)*

And do not take tranquilizers (unless a doctor has prescribed them for psychosis)! They are of no proven value in curing anything. They surely do not cure the cause of anxiety; rarely do they even truly ease it, and often they can bring on depression. Antidepressants, on the other hand, especially Elavil®, are often excellent, but only if they are really needed and only if taken for no longer than six months. Even here, at least 25 percent of patients can't take them because of complications.

You should be aware of the fact that physicians are relatively little influenced by the FDA-regulated drug package instructions.* It appears that common practice and perhaps pharmaceutical marketing encourage use outside that indicated on the "approved labeling." In three drugs tested, for instance, use was

---

*(George R. Mundy et al., "Current Medical Practice and the Food and Drug Administration," *JAMA* 229 (1974):1744–1748.

unorthodox from 57 percent to 78 percent of the time.
Moreover, investigation has shown that data on drug
complications is "incomplete, unrepresentative, uncontrolled."*

In the December 12, 1974, *New England Journal
of Medicine,* two tranquilizers—meprobamate (Mil-
town®) and chlordiazepoxide (Librium®)—were reported to show increases in congenital birth defects.
Valium® has had similar effects, with a 300 percent
increase in cleft palates. As an indication of how widespread their use is, Librium and Valium have made
their producer, Hoffmann-La Roche, the world's largest
drug manufacturer, making this company alone com-
parable in size with General Motors!

To get a flavor of how readily drugs can cause
complications, consider the warnings issued concerning
the antidepressant Nardil®:

Foods to avoid when on Nardil—

All cheeses except cottage cheese	Herring
	Nuts
Excessive amounts of caffeine and chocolate	Chopped liver
	Fresh baked breads
Vinegar, except white vinegar	Anything marinated
	Pods of broad beans
Anything fermented: yogurt, sour cream	Chicken livers

Liquors to avoid—

Beer	Gin
Dry red burgundy	Vodka
Bourbon	

Liquors you may have—

Rosé wines	Cordials
White wine, except sauterne	Scotch
Brandy	Rum

---

*Fred E. Karch and Louis Lasagna, "Adverse Drug Reactions,"
JAMA 234 (1975):1236–1241.

Do not take any other medications without a doctor's approval. That includes such common drugs as—
Contac®
Dristan®
Sinutabs

It so happens that Nardil, because of its numerous dangers, is not often prescribed, but consider Coumarin, a commonly used "blood thinner":

Drugs counteracting Coumarin—

Antacids	Chloral hydrate
Barbiturates	Griseofulvin (Fulvicin-
Glutethimide	U/F, Grifulvin V,
(Doriden®)	Grisactin®)
Meprobamate	Haloperidol (Haldol®)
(Equanil®, Miltown®)	Alcohol

Drugs enhancing Coumarin's effect—

Many antibiotics	Phenylbutazone
Chloramphenicol	(Butazolidin®)
(Chloromycetin®)	Oxyphenbutazone
Kanamycin sulfate	(Tandearil®)
(Kantrex®)	Indomethacin
Streptomycin sulfate	(Indocin®)
Sulfonamides	Aspirin
Tetracyclines	Diphenylhydantoin
Clofibrate	(Dilantin®)
(Atromid-S®)	Ethacrynic acid
	(Edecrin®)

Obviously, when you *do* need a drug you also need to look very carefully at everything else you ingest while you are taking it. Insist upon knowing *all* the precautions, warnings, and potential complications.

LIGHT

Dr. John Ott has done some truly remarkable work in the use of light. It appears that the human body, as well as plants and animals, requires a balance of the light spectrum found in natural daylight (or, should I say, *unpolluted* natural daylight)/People who are inside most of the day—at home or in an office—should insist on having full spectrum or daylight fluorescent lights overhead. In addition, everyone should try to be outside a minimum of two hours a day. That doesn't mean *looking* at the sun, of course, but just having the ambient daylight free to enter one's eyes unobstructed by glasses of any sort or any other impediment. For a very interesting and exciting discussion of light, I recommend Dr. Ott's book, *Health and Light*. Although this section on light is brief, the point is clearly made that its proper use is vital to the health of the total body.

MEDITATION

A great deal of work has been published and tremendous publicity has been accorded Transcendental Meditation (TM) in the past few years. Although TM *does* induce relaxation, its benefits have been almost exclusively in relation to the relaxation induced. TM has specifically failed to be of benefit in migraine headache patients and in chronic pain. Indeed, when we compare the extensive publications concerning TM with those on biofeedback, autogenic training, hypnosis, and progressive muscular relaxation, we find that TM rates fifth in effectiveness. *Anything TM can accomplish, all four of the others can do at least as well, without the need to join a semireligious cult.* (See table of Physiological Changes During Various Relaxation Techniques.)

Indeed, Dr. Herb Benson, who has done most of the clinical work with TM, has himself reported that one can do quite as well just breathing and repeating "one." For Westerners, "calm," "relaxed," and "serene" are more likely to be meaningful. Unfortunately, TM has a tendency to induce mindlessness or focusing on nothing.

Throughout recorded history, meditation has been a part of most religious philosophies. In its purest form, it is an attempt to attune oneself with the divine. Relaxation and physiological and emotional balancing are

PHYSIOLOGICAL CHANGES DURING VARIOUS RELAXATION TECHNIQUES

TECHNIQUE	OXYGEN CONSUMPTION	RATE OF RESPIRATION	PULSE RATE	ALPHA WAVES (EEG)	BLOOD PRESSURE	MUSCLE TENSION	CLINICAL EFFECTIVENESS IN TREATING SYMPTOMS AND DISEASES (IN DECREASING ORDER)
Biogenics: Biofeedback and autogenic training							2
Autogenic training							8
Progressive relaxation	?						3
Hypnosis					?		4
Zen and Yoga					in high BP	?	2
Transcendental Meditation					in high BP	?	5
Physical exercise	(during)	(during)	(during)	?	(by regular practice)		7

SUMMARY OF BIOGENICS TECHNIQUE

Autogenic Shift
Body Numb

Keep Well

Relaxation

Physiological balance

Altered State of Consciousness (Focusing)

As of now
Attention
Attentive

Get Well

Goals, programming

Physiological Mantra (Healing Phrase)

Visualization

Spiritual Attunement

Meditation

Attunement with God

prerequisites for meditation. Results are seldom satisfactory when meditation is attempted before one has the calmness that comes with regular mental balancing. Dr. J. H. Schultz, who originated autogenic training, emphasized that individuals should not try meditation until they had practiced the basic autogenic technique at least six months. You'll note that the regular, more comprehensive program we've outlined in this book leads to true meditation ability within three months. And meditation *is* the *going beyond* to the Divine.

The elaborate mental and physical exercise program I have presented in this book is safe, simple, and effective. When I have presented my work at dozens of workshops and about 100 meetings, it has been eagerly received. It is quite possible to follow the system entirely on your own. It will be even more fun if you make it a way of life for yourself and your family. Hopefully, someday the principles presented here will be taught in our schools. Until then, this work presents a holistic approach to life and health which you may constantly appreciate anew and expand as you practice. You create your own reality. Always work to create the condition desired. *Every thought is a prayer*. Think —pray—to the good, the beautiful, the true—to love.

Selected Bibliography

AMA News, Oct. 28, 1974.

Andersen, Marianne S., and Louis M. Savary. *Passages: A Guide for Pilgrims of the Mind.* New York: Harper & Row, 1972.

Assagioli, Roberto. *Psychosynthesis: A Manual of Principles and Techniques.* New York: The Viking Press, 1971.

Bailey, Alice A. *Esoteric Healing.* New York: Lucis Publishing Co., 1953.

Barber, Theodore X., Leo V. DiCara, Joe Kamiya, Neal E. Miller, David Shapiro, and Johann Stoyva, eds. *Biofeedback and Self-Control.* Chicago: Aldine-Atherton, Inc., 1971.

Benson, Herbert. *The Relaxation Response.* New York: William Morrow & Co., 1975.

Boyer, John J., and Fred W. Kasch. "Exercise Therapy in Hypertensive Men." *JAMA* 211 (1970): 1668–1671.

Brown, Barbara B. *New Mind, New Body Bio-Feedback: New Directions for the Mind.* New York: Harper & Row, 1974.

Castaneda, Carlos. *A Separate Reality.* New York: Pocket Books, 1972.

Cheraskin, E., and W. M. Ringsdorf, Jr., *Psychodietetics: Food as the Key to Emotional Health.* New York: Stein & Day, 1974.

Cooper, Kenneth. *Aerobics*. Philadelphia: J. B. Lippincott, 1968.

Diamond, Edwin. "Can Exercise Improve Your Brain Power?" *Readers Digest*, May 1973.

Feldenkrais, Moshe. *Awareness Through Movement: Health Exercises for Personal Growth*. New York: Harper & Row, 1972.

Freese, Arthur S. *Pain: The New Help for Your Pain*. New York: G. P. Putnam's Sons, 1974.

Friedman, Meyer, and Ray H. Rosenman. *Type A Behavior and Your Heart*. Greenwich, Conn.: Fawcett Publications, Inc., 1975.

Fromm, Erika, and Ronald E. Shor, eds. *Hypnosis: Research Developments and Perspectives*. Chicago: Aldine-Atherton, Inc., 1972.

Fuehs, Victor R. *Who Shall Live? Health, Economics and Social Choice*. New York: Basic Books, 1975.

Green, Elmer E., Alyce M. Green, and E. Dale Walters. "Voluntary Control of Internal States: Psychological and Physiological." *Journal of Transpersonal Psychology*, II (1970): 1–26.

Harris, Thomas A. *I'm OK—You're OK: A Practical Guide to Transactional Analysis*. New York: Harper & Row, 1967.

Hutschnecker, Arnold A. *The Will to Live*. New York: Cornerstone Library, 1972.

Jacobson, Edmund. *Progressive Relaxation*. Chicago: The University of Chicago Press, Midway Reprint, 1974.

Jensen, Ann, and Mary Lou Watkins. *Franz Anton Mesmer: Physician Extraordinaire*. New York: Garrett Publications, 1967.

Jung, C. G. *Mysterium Coniunctionis: An Inquiry into the Separation and Synthesis of Psychic Opposites in Alchemy*. London: Routledge and Kegan Paul, 1963.

———. *On the Nature of the Psyche*. Translated by R. F. C. Hull. Princeton, N.J.: Princeton University Press, 1969.

———. *Psyche and Symbol*. Edited by Violet S. deLaszlo. Garden City, N.Y.: Doubleday Anchor Books, 1958.

Karlins, Marvin, and Lewis M. Andrews. *Biofeedback: Turning on the Power of Your Mind*. New York: J. B. Lippincott, 1972.

Kroger, William S. *Clinical and Experimental Hypnosis: In Medicine, Dentistry and Psychology*. Philadelphia: J. B. Lippincott, 1963.

LaMott, Kenneth. *Escape from Stress*. New York: G. P. Putnam's Sons, 1974.

LeCron, Leslie M. *Self-Hypnotism: The Technique and Its Use in Daily Living.* Englewood Cliffs, N.J.: Prentice-Hall, Inc., 1971.

Lewis, Howard R., and Martha E. Lewis. *Psychosomatics: How Your Emotions Can Damage Your Health.* New York: The Viking Press, 1972.

Lindemann, Hannes. *Relieve Tension the Autogenic Way.* New York: Peter H. Wyden, 1974.

Lowen, Alexander. *The Betrayal of the Body.* New York: Collier Books, 1969.

Luthe, Wolfgang, and Johannes Schultz. *Autogenic Therapy.* 6 vol. New York: Grune & Stratton, 1969.

Maslow, A. H. *The Farther Reaches of Human Nature.* New York: The Viking Press, 1971.

Masters, Roy. *How Your Mind Can Keep You Well.* Los Angeles: Foundation Books, 1972.

McCamy, John C., and James Presley. *Human Life Styling: Keeping Whole in the Twentieth Century.* New York: Harper & Row, 1975.

Medical Tribune, Nov. 13, 1974.

Ornstein, Robert E. *The Psychology of Consciousness.* New York: The Viking Press, 1972.

Ostrander, Sheila, and Lynn Schroeder. *Psychic Discoveries Behind the Iron Curtain.* New York: Bantam Books, 1971.

Ott, John. *Health and Light: The Effects of Natural and Artificial Light on Man and Other Living Things.* Old Greenwich, Conn.: The Devin-Adair Company, 1973.

Oyle, Irving. *The Healing Mind.* Millbrae, Calif.: Celestial Arts, 1975.

Payne, Buryl. *Getting There Without Drugs.* New York: The Viking Press, 1973.

Prevention, Jan. 1976.

Sage, J. A. S. *Live to Be 100.* New York: Simon & Schuster, 1963.

Schechter, Paul J., et al.: "Sodium Chloride Preference in Essential Hypertension." *JAMA* 225 (1973): 1311–1315.

Schuller, Robert H. *Self-Love: The Dynamic Force of Success.* New York: Hawthorn Books, 1969.

Selye, Hans. *The Physiology and Pathology of Exposure to Stress.* Montreal: Acta, Inc., 1950.

———. *The Stress of Life.* New York: McGraw-Hill, 1956.

Smart, Allan. "Conscious Control of Physical and Mental States." *Menninger Foundation Perspective,* April–May, 1970.

Smiley, Emma M. *Not Guilty.* Los Angeles: Scrivener and Company, 1971.

Steadman, Alice. *Who's the Matter with Me?* Washington, D.C.: ESP Press, 1975.

Stevens, John O. *Awareness: Exploring, Experimenting, Experiencing.* New York: Bantam Books, 1973.

Tart, Charles T., ed. *Altered States of Consciousness.* New York: John Wiley & Sons, 1969.

Thommen, George. *Is This Your Day: How Biorhythm Helps You Determine Your Life Cycles.* New York: Crown Publishers, Inc., 1964.

Tournier, Paul. *Guilt and Grace: A Psychological Study.* Translated by Arthur W. Heathcote, New York: Harper & Row, 1962.

Watson, George. *Nutrition and Your Mind: The Psychochemical Response.* New York: Harper & Row, 1972.

Wolff, Harold G. *Stress and Disease.* Edited by Stewart Wolf and Helen Goodell. Springfield, Ill.: Charles C. Thomas, 1953.

Worrall, Ambrose. *Essay on Prayer.* Baltimore, 1952.

Index

ABOUT THE AUTHOR

C. NORMAN SHEALY, M.D., is the director of the Pain Rehabilitation Center in La Crosse, Wisconsin, and president of Biogenic Institutes, which teaches Biogenics techniques to professionals. He has also taught at Harvard, Case Western Reserve, the University of Wisconsin and the University of Minnesota medical schools, and is the author of *Occult Medicine Can Save Your Life: A Modern Doctor Looks at Unconventional Healing* and *The Pain Game.*

MS READ-a-thon–
a simple way
to start youngsters reading.

Boys and girls between 6 and 14 can join the MS READ-a-thon and help find a cure for Multiple Sclerosis by reading books. And they get two rewards—the enjoyment of reading, and the great feeling that comes from helping others.

Parents and educators: For complete information call your local MS chapter, or call toll-free (800) 243-6000. Or mail the coupon below.

Kids can help, too!

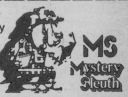

How's Your Health?

Bantam publishes a line of informative books, written by top experts to help you toward a healthier and happier life.

Bantam Book Catalog

Here's your up-to-the-minute listing of every book currently available from Bantam.

This easy-to-use catalog is divided into categories and contains over 1400 titles by your favorite authors.

So don't delay—take advantage of this special opportunity to increase your reading pleasure.

Just send us your name and address and 25¢ (to help defray postage and handling costs).